D1558487

Laparoscopic Surgery for Gynecologic Oncology

NOTICE

Laparoscopic Surgery for Gynecologic Oncology

Editors

Allan Covens, MD, FRCSC

Professor
Obstetrics and Gynecology
Gynecologic Oncology Site Group Leader
Toronto Sunnybrook Cancer Centre
Gynecologic Oncology Fellowship Director
University of Toronto
Toronto, Canada

Rachel Kupets, MD, MSc, FRCSC

Assistant Professor
Division of Gynecologic Oncology
Division of Surgical Oncology
Toronto Sunnybrook Regional Cancer Center
University of Toronto
Toronto, Canada

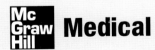
McGraw Hill **Medical**

New York   Chicago   San Francisco   Lisbon   London   Madrid   Mexico City   Milan
New Delhi   San Juan   Seoul   Singapore   Sydney   Toronto

Laparoscopic Surgery for Gynecologic Oncology

1 2 3 4 5 6 7 8 9 0   CTP/CTP   12 11 10 9 8

Set ISBN 978-0-07149324-6
Set MHID 0-07-149324-7
Book ISBN 978-0-07160624-0
Book MHID 0-07-160624-6
DVD ISBN 978-0-07160625-7
DVD MHID 0-07-160625-4

This book was set in Garamond by Aptara®, Inc.
The editors were Marsha Loeb, Christie Naglieri, and Lindsey Zahuranec.
The production supervisor was Sherri Souffrance.
Project management was provided by Satvinder Kaur, Aptara®, Inc.
The designer was Jonel Sofian. The cover designer is Pehrsson Design.
China Translation & Printing Service, Ltd., was printer and binder.

This book is printed on acid-free paper.

Library of Congress Cataloging-in-Publication Data

Laparoscopic surgery for gynecologic oncology / editors, Allan Covens,
    Rachel Kupets.—1st ed.
        p.   ;   cm.
    Includes bibliographical references and index.
    ISBN-13: 978-0-07-149324-6 (hardcover : alk. paper)
    ISBN-10: 0-07-149324-7 (hardcover : alk. paper)
    1. Generative organs, Female—Cancer—Endoscopic surgery.   I. Covens, Allan.
        II. Kupets, Rachel.
    [DNLM: 1. Genital Neoplasms, Female—surgery.   2. Laparoscopy—methods.
3. Gynecologic Surgical Procedures—methods. WP 145 L299 2009]
    RG104.7.L34   2009
    618.1′059—dc22

                                                                    2008014398

I would like to dedicate this book to my loving wife Pamela,
and children Louis, Stefanie, and Cari
who have put up with a frequent absent father most of their lives,
yet turned out to be terrific individuals.
Allan Covens, MD, FRCSC

To Polina, Paulina, and Madison—you have taught me that in life
anything is possible . . .
Rachel Kupets, MD, MSc, FRCSC

Contents

Contributors

Nadeem Abu-Rustum, MD
Associate Professor
Department of Surgical Oncology
Director
Minimally Invasive Surgery
Memorial Sloan-Kettering Cancer Center
New York, New York

Mario E. Beiner, MD
Staff
Department of Gynecologic Oncology and Pathology
The Chaim Sheba Medical Center
Tel Aviv University
Tel-Hashomer, Israel

Malik Boukerrou, MD
Staff
Department of Gynecologic Surgery
Jeanne de Flandre Hospital
University of Lille
Lille, France

David S. Bub, MD
Assistant Professor
Department of Surgery
Mount Sinai Medical School
New York, New York

M. Dwight Chen, MD
Staff Gynecologic Oncologist
Palo Alto Medical Clinic
El Camino Hospital
Mountain View, California

Dennis S. Chi, MD
Associate Professor
Department of Surgical Oncology
Director of Fellowship Program
Co-Director
Pelvic Reconstructive Surgery
Memorial Sloan-Kettering Cancer Center
New York, New York

Allan Covens, MD, FRCSC
Professor
Obstetrics and Gynecology
Gynecologic Oncology Site Group Leader
Toronto Sunnybrook Cancer Centre
Gynecologic Oncology Fellowship Director
University of Toronto
Toronto, Canada

Ram Eitan, MD
Staff
Division of Gynecologic Oncology
Tel Aviv University-Sackler School of Medicine
The Helen Schneider Hospital for Women
Rabin Medical Center
Petah-Tikva, Israel

Walid A. Farhat, MD
Associate Professor
Division of Urology
The Hospital for Sick Children
University of Toronto
Toronto, Ontario, Canada

Raja Flores, MD
Associate Professor
Department of Cardiothoracic Surgery
Weill Cornell Medical College
New York, New York

Jan Hauspy, MD
Assistant Professor
Division of Gynecologic Oncology
McMaster University
Juravinski Cancer Center
Hamilton, Ontario, Canada

Alayne Kealey, MD
Staff
Department of Anesthesia
Sunnybrook Health Sciences Center
University of Toronto
Toronto, Ontario, Canada

Siobhan M. Kehoe, MD
Fellow
Divison of Gynecologic Oncology
Memorial Sloan-Kettering Cancer Center
New York, New York

Lazar V. Klein, MD
Assistant Professor
Department of Surgery
University of Toronto
Division Head of Surgery
Humber River Regional Hospital
Toronto, Ontario, Canada

Rachel Kupets, MD, MSc, FRCSC
Assistant Professor
Division of Gynecologic Oncology
Division of Surgical Oncology
Toronto Sunnybrook Regional Cancer Center
University of Toronto
Toronto, Canada

Eric Lambaudie, MD
Staff
Department of Surgical Oncology
Paoli Calmettes Institute
Marseille, France

Eric Leblanc, MD
Professor and Head
Department Gynecologic Oncology
Oscar Lambret Cetner
Lille, France

Douglas A. Levine, MD
Staff
Department of Surgery
Memorial Sloan-Kettering Cancer Center
New York, New York

Katherine Moore, MD
Fellow
Division of Pediatric Urology
Hospital for Sick Children
University of Toronto
Toronto, Ontario, Canada

Nimesh P. Nagarsheth, MD
Assistant Professor
Division of Gynecologic Oncology
Mount Sinai School of Medicine
New York, New York

Fabrice Narducci, MD
Staff
Department of Gynecologic Surgery
Jeanne de Flandre Hospital
University of Lille
Lille, France

Farr Nezhat, MD
Professor and Chief Gynecologic Robotic
Minimally Invasive Programs
Head Fellowship Program
Division of Gynecologic Oncology
Mount Sinai Medical School
New York, New York

Katherine O'Hanlan, MD
Staff Gynecologic Oncologist
Gynecologic Oncology Associates
Sequoia Hospital
Portola Valley, California

Michele Peiretti, MD
Staff
Department of Gynecologic Oncology
European Institute of Oncology
Milan, Italy

Jerome Phalippou, MD
Staff
Department of Gynecologic Oncology
Oscar Lambert Center
Lille, France

Marie Plante, MD
Associate Professor and Chief
Division of Gynecologic Oncology
Laval University
Regional Hospital Center of Quebec
Quebec City, Canada

Denis Querleu, MD
Professor and Head
Institut Claudius Regaud
Cancer Center
University Paul-Sabatier
Toulouse, France

Pedro T. Ramirez, MD
Associate Professor
Director Minimally Invasive Surgery
Department of Gynecologic Oncology
University of Texas
MD Anderson Cancer Center
Houston, Texas

Michele Roy, MD
Professor
Department of Gynecologic Oncology
Laval University
Hotel-Dieu Regional Hospital Center
Quebec City, Quebec, Canada

Kathleen Schmeler, MD
Assistant Professor
Department of Gynecologic Oncology
University of Texas
MD Anderson Cancer Center
Houston, Texas

How To Use This Book

This book is meant as a learning tool for those interested in providing minimally invasive surgery to their patients with gynecologic cancers. This book may be used by fellows, residents, and staff people who desire to learn and fine-tune their operative skills.

This surgical textbook has a written component outlining the role of laparoscopy as well as a video component, which outlines the key set up and steps for these surgeries. Each chapter provides more than one video on a particular procedure so that the readers are exposed to different approaches, set up, techniques, and equipment that may be used to carry out the surgeries.

We are fortunate that some of the most recognized experts in this field have graciously donated their time and resources for the purpose of this book. With the aid of this book, gynecologic oncologists interested in minimally invasive surgery will benefit from the expert knowledge of our authors.

We hope that this book will serve as a great educational tool for many.

Allan Covens, MD, FRCSC
Rachel Kupets, MD, MSc, FRCSC

Preface

As minimally invasive surgery in gynecologic oncology grows and develops, patients and physicians alike are interested in its benefits to patient care and outcome. Those surgeons in the field are dedicated in providing laparoscopic surgery to their patients with gynecologic cancers. The purpose of this book is to serve as a learning tool for those in training as well as to those in practice who are committed to developing their laparoscopic surgical skills to their full potential.

This book is unique as it provides demonstrations by experts in the field of common gynecologic oncology laparoscopic procedures. Not only is there a didactic component to the book, but there is also a DVD section providing information on each procedure as well as a narration by the surgeon. The DVD component demonstrates more than one approach to performing common staging procedures so that the learner is made aware of options for set up, instrumentation, and technical aspects of the surgery.

We hope that this book will serve as an effective educational tool for those dedicated to providing women with gynecologic cancers the best possible surgical care.

And now, on to the book. . . .

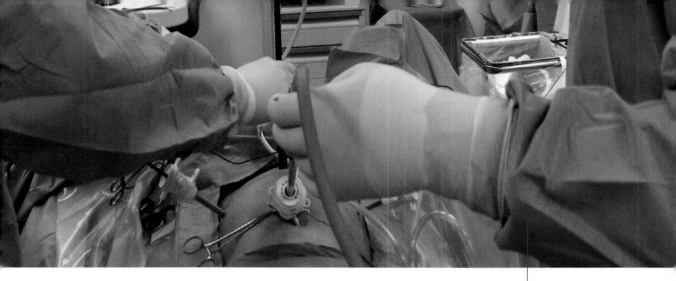

THE ROLE OF LAPAROSCOPY IN GYNECOLOGIC ONCOLOGY

1

Rachel Kupets and Allan L. Covens

Minimally invasive surgery has become a key component of care in gynecologic oncology. With the advancements in laparoscopic equipment such as the harmonic scalpel, the ligasure device, suturing instruments, endostaplers, and argon equipment, laparoscopy in gynecologic care has broadened from being a diagnostic tool to enabling gynecologic oncologists to perform extensive operative procedures.

Laparoscopy in gynecologic oncology has progressed from procedures such as a laparoscopically assisted vaginal hysterectomy to many more complex procedures such as total abdominal simple and radical hysterectomies, pelvic and aortic node dissection, omentectomy, and advanced bowel surgery.

A recent survey of the Society of Gynecologic Oncologists has indicated that its members believe in the benefits of laparoscopy for their patients.[1] It is certain that minimally invasive surgery will become increasingly offered to patients as training programs evolve to teach its trainees laparoscopic skills.

Minimally invasive surgery has a role in the surgical management of all disease sites treated by gynecologic oncologists.

ROLE OF LAPAROSCOPY IN CERVICAL CANCER

Credit must be given to Daniel Dargent for pioneering radical vaginal hysterectomy combined with laparoscopic pelvic lymphadenectomy. Since then, other surgeons have reported on their experiences. A comparison between laparoscopic-assisted radical vaginal hysterectomy and radical abdominal hysterectomy indicated that early cervical cancer may be treated by either route with similar efficacy and recurrence rates. The benefit of the minimally invasive approach included less intraoperative blood loss and shorter hospital stay by a median difference of 4 days.[2]

Spirtos et al.[3] published his outcomes on 78 patients with early cervical cancer who underwent laparoscopic total radical hysterectomies with pelvic and aortic lymph node dissections. He described his technique using the argon beam coagulator and endoscopic staplers. He was able to complete the cases laparoscopically in all but five cases. The average operating time was 205 minutes, average blood loss was 225 mL, and average lymph node count was 34 nodes. The transfusion rate was 1.3%, one patient developed a ureterovaginal fistula, and three patients had intraoperative cystotomies of which two were repaired laparoscopically.

Abu-Rustum et al.[4] also published their data on total laparoscopic radical hysterectomy with the argon beam coagulator. The authors were successful in completing their cases laparoscopically 90% of the time. The authors also reported that the blood loss was significantly less in the laparoscopic arm than a historic laparotomy arm; length of hospital stay was also significantly less in the minimally invasive arm.

Nezhat et al.[5] and Ramirez et al.[6] also reported on their institutional outcomes for total laparoscopic radical hysterectomies and pelvic lymphadenectomies. The authors reported acceptable nodal counts, clear margins, very low transfusion rate, and short hospital stays of 1 to 3 days on average.

ROLE OF LAPAROSCOPY IN OVARIAN CANCER

Childers et al.[7] were among the first to describe the feasibility of laparoscopic surgical staging of ovarian cancer. Since then, other centers have reported on their experiences. Tozzi et al.[8] reported on 24 patients who were either primarily staged or reoperated on after an initial procedure diagnosed cancer of the ovary. The staging included pelvic and para-aortic lymphadenectomies, appendectomies, and omentectomies. Of the 24 patients, 5 were upstaged and received chemotherapy and no major intra-operative complications occurred.

Chi et al.[9] performed a case control study comparing outcomes of patients staged for ovarian cancer with laparoscopy or laparotomy. They found no difference in the adequacy of surgical specimen including nodal count and size of omental specimen.

Leblanc et al.[10] reported on 53 patients with clinical stage I disease who were restaged laparoscopically. Of these, 42 patients were restaged after the primary operation while 11 underwent chemotherapy first. Mean operating time was 238 minutes; average nodes retrieved were 20 aortic nodes and 14 pelvic nodes, respectively. Hospital stay ranged from 1 to 5 days. Complications included epigastric vessel injury, lymphocysts, and ureteric transaction in one case. Nineteen percent of the patients were upstaged, mostly from positive aortic and pelvic nodes and none developed port site metastases.

Abu-Rustum et al.[11] also reported on the utility of laparoscopy as a second look procedure for epithelial ovarian cancer. Comparing laparoscopy to a laparotomy arm through a retrospective chart review, he determined that the minimally invasive approach was feasible, provided the same information as a laparotomy. Patients had shorter procedures and hospital stays.

Littell et al.[12] reported on patients in phase II clinical trials who underwent second look laparoscopies when deemed to have had a clinical clinical response (CR). Those patients who had a negative laparoscopy went on to have a laparotomy. The study calculated that the negative predictive value of a negative second look laparoscopy is 91% with a sensitivity of 85%.

ROLE OF LAPAROSCOPY IN PELVIC AND PARA–AORTIC LYMPH NODE DISSECTION

Extensive lymph node dissection is key to the surgical management for all gynecologic malignancies. Daniel Dargent was the first to report on laparoscopic lymphadenectomy in 1989.

Querleu et al.[13] was the next to report on the technique for laparoscopic pelvic lymphadenectomy in early cervical cancer.

Nezhat et al.[14] was the first to report on the technique of laparoscopic para-aortic lymph node dissection in 1992.

Since these initial reports, many centers have reported on their experiences in extensive lymph node sampling. Scribner et al.[15] reported on 100 cases of pelvic and para-aortic lymphadenectomies performed laparoscopically for endometrial and ovarian cancers. These surgeons were able to retrieve on average 18 aortic nodes and 7 pelvic nodes. Complications included one cystotomy, one ureteric injury, two pulmonary embolisms, six wound infections, and bowel herniation through a trocar site. One death occurred from vascular injury to the internal iliac vein and second perioperative death was caused by a pulmonary embolism. The main reasons for conversion to laparotomy included obesity with a 30% conversion rate, previous adhesions with a 17% conversion rate and intraperitoneal disease.

Since these initial reports, many centers have reported on the feasibility and safety of laparascopic pelvic and aortic lymphadenectomy.[16–18]

ROLE OF LAPAROSCOPY IN ENDOMETRIAL CANCER

Surgery for endometrial cancer ranges from laparoscopically assisted vaginal hysterectomies (LAVH) to total laparoscopic hysterectomies (TLH) and lymph node survey. Surgeons are becoming more interested in the TLH approach whose benefit includes ability to directly see all anatomic structures as well as no need for uterine prolapse.

Ghezzi et al.[19] reported on a small randomized trial comparing LAVH to TLH in endometrial cancer; patients also underwent pelvic node dissections. The group reported a shorter operating time in the TLH group by 40 minutes and less intraoperative complications. Port site metastases and vaginal metastases were not increased in the TLH group.

Obermair also performed a retrospective review comparing a laparoscopic total abdominal hysterectomy to open hysterectomy. The patterns of recurrence were similar in both groups and no port site metastases were noted in the TLH arm. The method of surgery did not impact the disease free or overall survival.[20]

The largest randomized to trial comparing laparoscopic management of endometrial cancer to traditional open surgery was the GOG LAP-2 trial. A total of 2616 patients were enrolled into the study, among them, 920 received a laparotomy while 1696 were randomized to laparoscopy. There was a 23% conversion rate to laparotomy in the scope arm. Length of hospital stay was shorter in the laparoscopy arm by a difference of 1 day on average while the operating time was longer by 1 hour on average. Survival data has yet to be reported on this study. The results of the study were presented at the Society of Gynecologic Oncologists annual meeting (2006), Palm Springs, California, USA.

ROLE OF LAPAROSCOPY AND PELVIC EXENTERATION

As the role of laparoscopy is expanding in gynecologic oncology there have been reports of its utility in evaluating exenteration candidates. Plante and Roy[21] reported on three patients who were evaluated laparoscopically to determine site of recurrent disease. There were no intraoperative complications and they were able to select their candidates appropriately.

Kohler et al.[22] reported on their experiences with laparoscopy prior to exenteration on 41 patients. The authors were able to select out patients eligible for exenteration and determined that laparoscopy did not miss any pathology that was subsequently detected during the exenteration laparotomy. They were able to successfully detect recurrent disease which prevented those patients from undergoing an unnecessary laparotomy.

ROLE OF LAPAROSCOPY IN THE OBESE AND OLDER ADULTS

While a challenging prospect, laparoscopy has been successfully carried out in obese patients. Eltabbakh et al.[23] reported on the feasibility and safety of laparoscopy in obese women with endometrial cancer. The study prospectively collected data on women whose BMI ranged from 28 to 60 and compared those outcomes to a control group of women of similar BMI who underwent laparotomy in the 2 years prior. Laparoscopic surgery was successfully completed in 88% of patients. Although laparoscopic surgery took longer than open, the surgeons were able to retrieve more pelvic lymph nodes, patients had less blood loss, less postoperative pain, and shorter hospital stay. Scribner et al.[24] reported on feasibility of performing laparoscopic pelvic and para-aortic lymph node dissection in obese women of a Quetelet index (QI) ≥ 28 these outcomes were compared to a historic control arm of patients undergoing laparotomy. Laparoscopy was successfully completed in 64% of the 55 patients. A QI of ≥ 35 tended to be more likely to be converted to laparotomy with an 82% conversion rate. As compared to the historic laparotomy arm, patients who underwent laparoscopy had similar blood loss and transfusion rates and length of hospital stay was significantly shorter.

O'Hanlan et al.[25] and Eisenhauer et al.[26] reported on their experiences in performing laparoscopic hysterectomies in obese patients in their respective sites. O'Hanlan et al.[25] reported on a 4.5% complication rate which included only ureteric injury, laparotomy for bleeding, and an incisional hernia. Eisenhauer et al.[26] reported on superior node counts in obese patients undergoing laparoscopic staging for uterine cancer as compared to patients undergoing laparotomy.

Scribner et al.[24,27] reported on laparoscopic management of early stage endometrial cancer in the older adults defined as ≥65 years. The authors determined that in their series of 67 patients undergoing laparoscopic surgery, there were a shorter length of stay, less postoperative fevers, less postoperative ileus and fewer wound complications.

QUALITY OF LIFE AND LAPAROSCOPIC SURGERY

Two trials have set out to prospectively evaluate quality of life outcomes in patients undergoing minimally invasive surgery. The LACE trial was designed to assess quality of life outcomes in patients undergoing a total laparoscopic approach in the treatment of endometrial cancer as compared to laparotomy. The results are pending.[28]

The GOG LAP-2 study also had a quality of life component. The results indicate that for women having undergone laparoscopic hysterectomy, salpingooherectomy, pelvic and aortic node dissections, as compared to those with open procedures, had a better overall quality of life, physical functioning, personal appearance, and an earlier resumption to normal activities than did the laparotomy patients. At 6 months, there were no quality of life differences between the two surgeries, with the exception of laparoscopy patients reporting better body image than the laparotomy patients.[29]

CONCLUSION

Operative techniques in gynecologic oncology have been adapted to lend themselves to a laparoscopic approach. There is no doubt that laparoscopy has a key role in management of women with early gynecologic malignancies. The operative techniques are feasible, safe, and effective. While laparoscopy offers the same information on staging, as does conventional surgery, it provides a rapid recovery and discharge from the hospital, which are desirable by both patient and physician. There is willingness and desire by gynecologic oncologists to offer minimally invasive surgical options to their patients, while at the same time patient demand is also on the rise.

This book will serve as an important educational tool for those who wish to learn laparoscopy in gynecologic oncology.

REFERENCES

1. Frumovitz M, Ramirez PT, Greer M, et al. Laparoscopic training and practice in gynecologic oncology among Society of Gynecologic Oncologists members and fellows-in-training. *Gynecol Oncol.* 2004;94(3):746–753.

2. Steed H, Rosen B, Murphy J, et al. A comparison of laparascopic-assisted radical vaginal hysterectomy and radical abdominal hysterectomy in the treatment of cervical cancer. *Gynecol Oncol.* 2004;93(3):588–593.

3. Spirtos NM, Eisenkop SM, Schlaerth JB, Ballon SC. Laparoscopic radical hysterectomy (type III) with aortic and pelvic lymphadenectomy in patients with stage I cervical cancer: Surgical morbidity and intermediate follow-up. *Am J Obstet Gynecol.* 2002;187(2):340–348.

4. Abu-Rustum NR, Chi DS, Sonoda Y, et al. Total laparoscopic radical hysterectomy with pelvic lymphadenectomy using the argon-beam coagulator: Pilot data and comparison to laparotomy. *Gynecol Oncol.* 2003;91(2):402–409.

5. Nezhat F, Mahdavi A, Nagarsheth NP. Total laparoscopic radical hysterectomy and pelvic lymphadenectomy using harmonic shears. *J Minim Invasive Gynecol.* 2006;13(1):20–25.

6. Ramirez PT, Slomovitz BM, Soliman PT, et al. Total laparoscopic radical hysterectomy and lymphadenectomy: The M. D. Anderson Cancer Center experience. *Gynecol Oncol.* 2006;102(2):252–255.

7. Childers JM, Lang J, Surwit EA, Hatch KD. Laparoscopic surgical staging of ovarian cancer. *Gynecol Oncol.* 1995;59(1):25–33.

8. Tozzi R, Köhler C, Ferrara A, Schneider A. Laparoscopic treatment of early ovarian cancer: Surgical and survival outcomes. *Gynecol Oncol.* 2004;93(1):199–203.

9. Chi DS, Abu-Rustum NR, Sonoda Y, et al. The safety and efficacy of laparoscopic surgical staging of apparent stage I ovarian and fallopian tube cancers. *Am J Obstet Gynecol.* 2005;192(5):1614–1619.

10. Leblanc E et al. Laparoscopic restaging of early stage invasive adnexal tumors: A 10-year experience. *Gynecol Oncol.* 2004;94(3):624–629.

11. Abu-Rustum NR, Barakat RR, Siegel PL, et al. Second-look operation for epithelial ovarian cancer: Laparoscopy or laparotomy? *Obstet Gynecol.* 1996;88(4 Pt 1): 549–553.

12. Littell RD, Hallonquist H, Matulones U, et al. Negative laparoscopy is highly predictive of negative second-look laparotomy following chemotherapy for ovarian, tubal, and primary peritoneal carcinoma. *Gynecol Oncol.* 2006;103(2):570–574.

13. Querleu D, Leblanc E, and Castelain B. Laparoscopic pelvic lymphadenectomy in the staging of early carcinoma of the cervix. *Am J Obstet Gynecol.* 1991; 164(2):579–581.

14. Nezhat CR, Mahdavi A, Nagarseth NP, et al. Laparoscopic radical hysterectomy with paraaortic and pelvic node dissection. *Am J Obstet Gynecol.* 1992;166(3): 864–865.

15. Scribner DR, Jr., Walker JL, Johnson GA, et al. Laparoscopic pelvic and paraaortic lymph node dissection: Analysis of the first 100 cases. *Gynecol Oncol.* 2001;82(3): 498–503.

16. Abu-Rustum NR, Chi DS, Sonoda Y, et al. Transperitoneal laparoscopic pelvic and para-aortic lymph node dissection using the argon-beam coagulator and monopolar instruments: An 8-year study and description of technique. *Gynecol Oncol.* 2003;89(3):504–513.

17. Dottino PR, Tobias DH, Beddoe A, et al. Laparoscopic lymphadenectomy for gynecologic malignancies. *Gynecol Oncol.* 1999;73(3):383–388.

18. Kohler C, Tozzi R, Klemm P, Schneider A. Laparoscopic paraaortic left-sided transperitoneal infrarenal lymphadenectomy in patients with gynecologic malignancies: Technique and results. *Gynecol Oncol.* 2003;91(1):139–148.

19. Ghezzi F, Cromi A, Uccella S, et al. Laparoscopy versus laparotomy for the surgical management of apparent early stage ovarian cancer. *Gynecol Oncol.* 2007;105(2): 409–413.

20. Obermair A, Manolitsas TP, Leung Y, Hammond IG, McCartney AJ. Total laparoscopic hysterectomy for endometrial cancer: Patterns of recurrence and survival. *Gynecol Oncol.* 2004;92(3):789–793.

21. Plante M, Roy M. The use of operative laparoscopy in determining eligibility for pelvic exenteration in patients with recurrent cervical cancer. *Gynecol Oncol.* 1995;59(3):401–404.

22. Köhler C, Tozzi R, Possover M, Schneider A. Explorative laparoscopy prior to exenterative surgery. *Gynecol Oncol.* 2002;86(3):311–315.

23. Eltabbakh GH, Shamonki MI, Moody JM, Garafano LL. Hysterectomy for obese women with endometrial cancer: Laparoscopy or laparotomy? *Gynecol Oncol.* 2000;78(3 Pt 1):329–335.

24. Scribner DR Jr, Walker JL, Johnson GA, et al. Laparoscopic pelvic and paraaortic lymph node dissection in the obese. *Gynecol Oncol.* 2002;84(3):426–430.

25. O'Hanlan KA, Dibble SL, Fisher DT. Total laparoscopic hysterectomy for uterine pathology: Impact of body mass index on outcomes. *Gynecol Oncol.* 2006;103(3):938–941.

26. Eisenhauer EL, Wypych KA, Mehrara BJ, et al. Comparing surgical outcomes in obese women undergoing laparotomy, laparoscopy, or laparotomy with panniculectomy for the staging of uterine malignancy. *Ann Surg Oncol.* 2007;14(8): 2384–2391.

27. Scribner DR Jr, Walker JL, Johnson GA, et al. Surgical management of early-stage endometrial cancer in the elderly: Is laparoscopy feasible? *Gynecol Oncol.* 2001;83(3):563–568.

28. Zullo F, Palomba S, Russo T, et al. A prospective randomized comparison between laparoscopic and laparotomic approaches in women with early stage endometrial cancer: A focus on the quality of life. *Am J Obstet Gynecol.* 2005;193(4):1344–1352.

29. Annual Meeting on Women's Cancer, March 2006. Palm Springs, California.

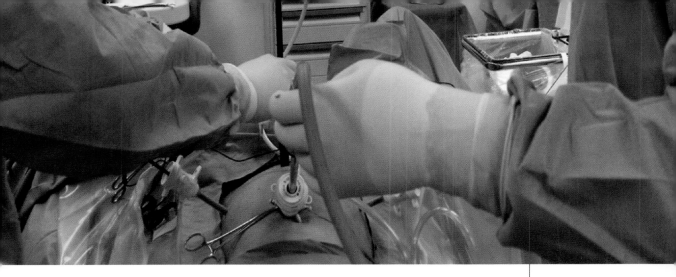

TOTAL LAPAROSCOPIC HYSTERECTOMY | 2

Siobhan M. Kehoe, Douglas A. Levine, and
Nadeem R. Abu-Rustum

INTRODUCTION

Minimally invasive surgery has been utilized in the field of gynecology for many decades and was introduced into gynecologic oncology in the 1990s. Laparoscopic pelvic and para-aortic lymph node dissection for endometrial cancer was described by Childers and Surwit[1] in 1992. Laparoscopy has been shown to be feasible and beneficial in select gynecologic oncology patients. Complex gynecologic oncology procedures can be performed with a low rate of complication and minimal morbidity. Laparoscopy is being incorporated into multiple areas within the field of gynecologic oncology and currently, advanced laparoscopic techniques are used to treat cervical, endometrial, and ovarian malignancies. While these complicated procedures can result in increased operative times, the benefits include decreased postoperative pain as well as shorter postoperative recovery time with a shorter length of hospital stay.

The laparoscopic hysterectomy (LH) involves performing the hysterectomy and specifically the ligation of the uterine arteries through the laparoscope. With this approach, the uterus and adnexa can still be removed through the vagina and the completion of the surgery (closure of the vaginal cuff) can be performed vaginally. The laparoscopic-assisted vaginal hysterectomy (LAVH), described by Reich et al.[2] in 1989, involves ligating the round ligaments and ovarian vessels laparoscopically and then performing a vaginal hysterectomy and ligation of the uterine arteries through the vaginal route. Alternatively, a total laparoscopic hysterectomy (TLH) is defined as ligation of all intraperitoneal ligaments and vascular pedicles, including the uterine arteries, laparoscopically with no vaginal surgery being performed. In a TLH, the uterus can be removed vaginally but the vaginal cuff is then re-approximated with laparoscopically placed sutures. Therefore, TLH means the entire procedure is completed laparoscopically. This chapter will focus specifically on the technique of TLH.

The technique of TLH can vary between institutions and surgeons. There are multiple types of instruments such as energy sources and cauterization devices that can be used to perform this procedure. At the same time, while the basic steps of the procedure remain constant, slight alterations in these steps such as the uterine artery ligation or closure of the vaginal cuff can be seen. This chapter will review the steps of a TLH and identify different instruments that can be used to perform a TLH.

| INDICATIONS/CONTRAINDICATIONS

Before reviewing the procedure, it is important to understand some general concepts about laparoscopy before proceeding. One of the most important points of laparoscopy is learning which patients are the best candidates for this approach. There are straightforward factors that help determine whether laparoscopy would be appropriate and successful for your patient. Patient characteristics including history of prior surgeries and weight are important. Attempting laparoscopy in patients with prior surgeries is acceptable but conversion may be necessary if the adhesions are too dense and exposure is compromised.

Obesity is not a contraindication to laparoscopy as many series have reported successful procedures in the obese population.[3–6] Areas of difficulty with laparoscopy in the obese patient include the entrance into the peritoneal cavity and obtaining exposure and visualization within the abdominal and pelvic cavities. This factor may be more of a hindrance in completing other laparoscopic procedures such as pelvic or para-aortic lymphadenectomy. Conversion to laparotomy may be warranted if exposure is limited because of the size of the patient. Obermair et al. compared TLH and TAH in obese women with endometrial cancer. TLH was successfully completed in 89.4% of the patients. Wound infections occurred in 2.1% in the TLH group compared to 48.4% in the TAH group.[3] Eltabbakh et al. reported a 7.5% conversion rate in a series of 40 obese women undergoing LAVH for endometrial cancer. Those women who completed the LAVH had a shorter recovery period and returned to full activity and work sooner than those undergoing TAH.[4] A significant benefit of laparoscopy is the lower rate of postoperative wound infection which is often a major complication after laparotomy in the obese.

The size of the uterus is also an important factor since for oncologic procedures the uterus must be removed intact. There is not an exact overall size of the uterus that is defined as a contraindication for laparoscopic gynecologic surgery. However, an arbitrary cut-off size has been reported suggesting that a minimally invasive surgical gynecologic procedure would not be recommended. This size is greater than 8 cm in the width of the fundus or lower uterine segment on CT scan since this may limit the lateral dissection and this size uterus may not be able to be removed from the vagina without morcellation. Also, the extent of disease and spread of cancer to other organs will need to be assessed in order to determine if the procedure can adequately be performed and completed laparoscopically.

There is a definite learning curve for laparoscopic procedures. Surgeon skill and comfort level must be considered as one weighs the surgical options for treating the patient. This may be another factor in the decision-making process for which cases to proceed with laparoscopy.

TECHNIQUE

Set-up, patient positioning, and equipment

A key to a successful laparoscopic procedure is preparing for a laparoscopic case. Therefore, set-up of the room including appropriate positioning of the patient, lights, video screens, and power supply tower is important. In order to proceed with the procedure, there should be functioning monitors/screens for the surgeon and all assistants. The power sources should be functioning and the insufflation device should have sufficient CO_2 gas. It is also crucial to have appropriate and functioning instruments. The instruments used may vary depending on what is available at your institution. Some of the necessary instruments include 5- and 12-mm trocars, a coagulation device, a monopolar instrument, a vaginal probe, irrigation and suction device, and laparoscopic suturing devices.[7] Some of the most common coagulation devices include the argon beam coagulator (ABC) (CONMED Endoscopic Tech, MA, USA), the Harmonic Scalpel (Ethicon Endo-Surgery, Cincinnati, OH, USA), and the LigaSure (Valleylab, Boulder, CO, USA). The ABC can be used as a coagulator and a dissector, while the Harmonic Scalpel and the LigaSure can coagulate and ligate.

The patient is placed in the supine position on the operating table. Lower extremity compression devices are placed on the patient for venous thrombosis prophylaxis prior to induction of anesthesia. General endotracheal anesthesia is administered and an orogastric or nasogastric tube should be placed to decompress the stomach.

The Allen stirrups are set up on the operating table and the patient is placed in the dorsolithotomy position. The patient should be moved down on the table so that the uterine manipulator can be moved in all directions. It is important to assess the positioning of the legs within the stirrups. The height of the stirrup is altered to reduce strain or compression of the inguinal region to avoid injury to the nerve. The hip should not be minimally flexed and this can be achieved by aligning the knee with the iliac crest and toward the direction of the contralateral shoulder. The weight of the leg should be on the heel in the base of the boot. There should be minimal to no weight on the back of the knee and calf to decrease pressure on the peroneal nerve. The patient's arms should be tucked alongside her body to allow the surgeons ability to move without restriction. Generally, a rolled pad is placed within the patient's hands and the arms are generously wrapped with pads for protection when the table or legs are moved. It is important to be cautious of IV access and O_2 monitors when tucking the arms (Figure 2-1).

At this point the patient is prepped (including the abdomen, perineum, and vagina) and draped in the normal fashion. The vaginal setup must be performed before the laparoscopic procedure can commence. A foley catheter should be placed in the bladder to allow for drainage before trocars are inserted. Then, a sterile speculum is placed in the vagina and the anterior portion of the cervix is grasped with a tenaculum. The uterus is sounded for size and then the cervix is only minimally dilated to allow the tight placement of a uterine manipulator. Either a disposable and reusable uterine manipulators can be used. There are multiple types of uterine manipulator including the Valthcev, the Pelosi, the HUMI, and the disposable manipulator.

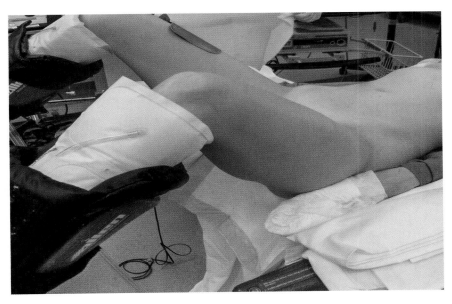

Figure 2-1 ■ Patient positioning.
The picture shows the patient in the dorsolithotomy position with the legs in Allen stirrups. Notice that the arms are wrapped and placed alongside the body.

Before commencing the procedure, the anatomical landmarks should be assessed on the patient. The umbilicus is at the level of L3 and L4 while the bifurcation of the aorta is between L4 and L5. The relationship between the umbilicus and the iliac crests is established. In general, four ports are used in most gynecologic cancer laparoscopic procedures. The initial 12-mm port is placed in the umbilicus and for the most part is the trocar which holds the camera. A 12-mm suprapubic port and two 5-mm lateral ports are used for surgical instruments to perform the procedure. The patient should be kept horizontal in the supine position without any Trendelenburg at this point.

The surgeon is positioned on the left side of the patient while the first assistant is at the right side and a second assistant can stand between the legs. Each surgeon must have a monitor/screen in front of them and adjusted to their comfort (Figure 2-2). The tower which holds the light source for the camera and the insufflation box which supplies the air and monitors the pressure should be positioned close to the patient (Figure 2-3).

There are a number of ways to approach the entrance in the umbilicus including the open technique, direct trocar insertion or the transumbilical

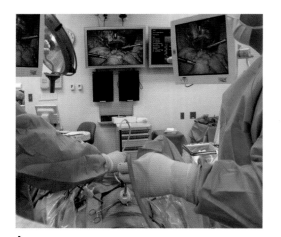

A

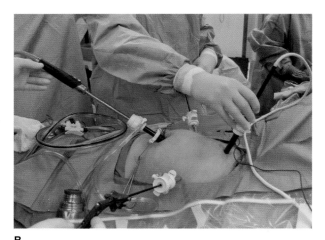

B

Figure 2-2 ▪ Position of surgeons.
A. Position of surgeons in relation to patient and monitors. The primary surgeon is positioned on the left side and uses the video screen on the right. B. Note that the surgeon should be in a comfortable position with the height of the table adjusted to allow for manipulation of the instruments.

insertion of a Veress needle. Other methods of insufflation include transuterine insertion of a Veress needle or left upper quadrant Veress needle insertion. Entrance into the abdominal cavity, obtaining a pneumoperitoneum and placement of the trocar are critical steps in the laparoscopic procedure.

We begin by placing the umbilical port using the open technique in all cases in order to reduce risk of vascular injury. The initial incision is made infraumbilically. If there is an infraumbilical hernia or if body habitus limits the ability to enter below the umbilicus, the incision and trocar can be placed supraumbilically. Using a 10-blade scalpel, a 1 to 2 cm vertical incision is made below the umbilicus. Using S-shaped retractors to expose, the incision is extended sharply down to the fascia. The fascia is grasped with clamps, elevated and entered sharply with knife or scissors. The major point is to continue to elevate while making incisions in order to reduce the risk of injuring the bowel. Once the fascia is entered and confirmed, the peritoneum can be incised. The fascial edges are tagged with two 2-O absorbable sutures. A 10- or 12-mm trocar with a blunt obturator is then placed into the abdominal cavity and is secured in place using the fascial anchoring sutures (Figure 2-4).

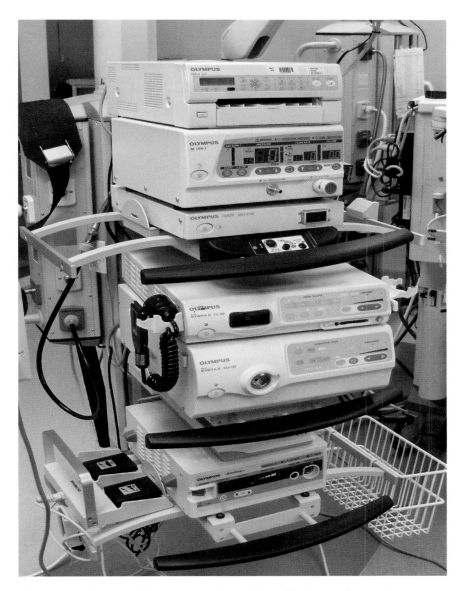

Figure 2-3 ▪ **Tower with power supply and insufflation equipment.**

Insufflation of the abdomen can then take place using this umbilical port. Initially the gas flow is set to 30 L/min to allow for a fast flow rate into the abdomen. The pressure is left at 12–15 mm Hg and is not to exceed this pressure throughout the surgery. A 0-degree laparoscope is placed in through this port and the abdomen and pelvis are inspected in order

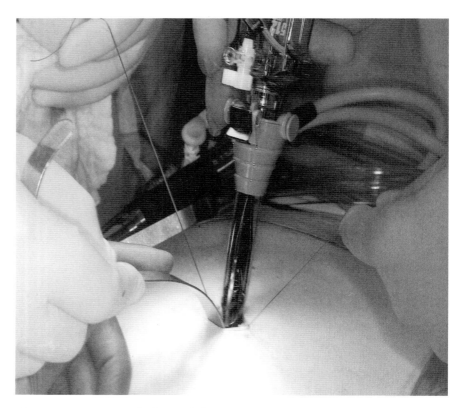

Figure 2-4 ▪ Open technique of abdominal entry.
The open technique is one method of initial trocar placement. This technique can help to decrease vascular injury with entrance into the abdominal cavity. Two sutures on the fascia allow the trocar to be kept in place. These two sutures also help identify the fascia for closure at the end of the case.

to assess extent of disease and adhesions. It is important at this point to take a moment to assess if the procedure should be continued laparoscopically.

After one decides to proceed laparoscopically, the right and left lower lateral ports can be inserted. The inferior epigastric blood vessels located in the lateral umbilical fold of the abdominal wall can and should be visualized with the laparoscope. Then a 1-cm skin incision is made approximately 2 fingerbreadths medial and caudal to the iliac crest to avoid vascular injury. A 5-mm trocar is inserted under direct visualization (the same procedure is performed on the right and left). A 12-mm trocar will also be placed midline suprapubically to aid in dissection and manipulation.

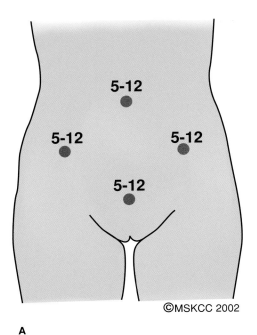

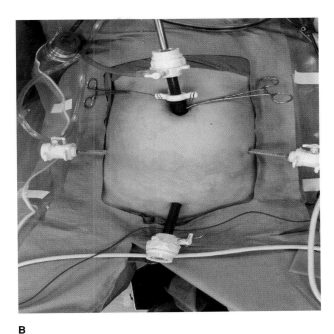

©MSKCC 2002

A   B

Figure 2-5 ▪ Abdominal placement of trocars.
A. Schematic representation of one type of final trocar placements. The complex gynecologic procedures require four ports. The two lateral ports are 5 mm and can be used
for most instruments. The suprapubic port is generally a larger port (10–12 mm) and
the larger instruments including the ABC, endoscopic stapler or the LigaSure can be
placed through this port. (Reproduced with permission from Medical Graphics, Memorial Sloan-Kettering Cancer Center.) B. This is the final port placement in a patient with
four disposable trocars placed in the abdomen. Disposable or reusable trocars can be
used.

Again, a 1-cm incision is made 2 to 3 cm above the symphysis pubis. Visu-
alizing the lower abdominal wall and the location of the bladder can help
direct where the incision should be and with the direct placement of the
midline port. The final trocar arrangement is shown in Figure 2-5.

Total laparoscopic hysterectomy

Generally, inspection and identification of pelvic structures is easiest when
the patient is placed in steep Trendelenberg. The bowels are mobilized
into the upper abdomen to allow for visualization. Identification of the
ureters is crucial before beginning the procedure. The ureters can be
found by different approaches. The uterus can be elevated with the

manipulator to gain better exposure. The ureter can usually be identified at its entrance into the pelvis and can be followed along the pelvic sidewall.

The first step is to ligate the round ligaments laterally. This can be performed with a number of instruments including the LigaSure, the ABC or another coagulation device such as the monopolar cautery. The round ligament needs to be completely divided as the artery of Sampson runs just beneath the round ligament and may cause bleeding if not cauterized before ligation. The LigaSure is a sealing device which can be used to cauterize and ligate vessels. The ABC is useful as it can be used as an energy source as well as a dissector. The ABC helps achieve hemostasis while performing the division of the round ligament and its adjacent vessels.

The Harmonic ACE ultrasonic device can also be used for vessel sealing and ligating. These devices allow for minimal thermal spread which is important during this procedure because of the proximity to the ureters. An important fact to remember is that the round ligament should be placed on traction when being divided (Figure 2-6). An important key to any

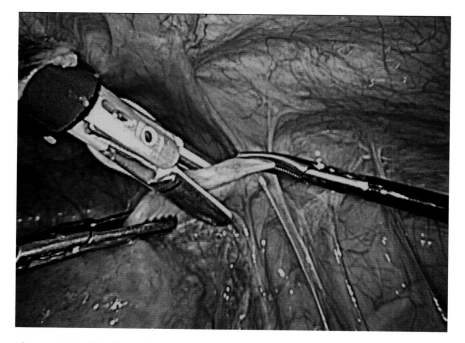

Figure 2-6 ■ Ligation of the round ligament with the LigaSure.
The round ligament is placed on tension with opposing laparoscopic instruments. It is then cauterized and transected.

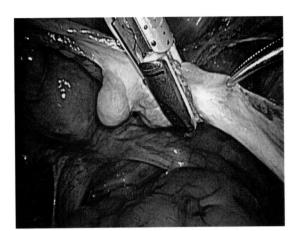

A

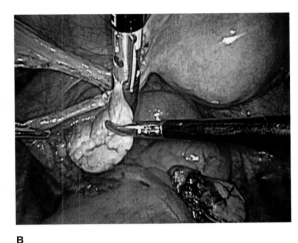

B

Figure 2-7 ▪ **Isolation and ligation of the ligament.**
A. Isolation and ligation of the IP ligament. Many patients will undergo a bilateral salpingo-oophorectomy in conjunction with the TLH. In these patients, the IP ligament is isolated and then ligated. Here the IP ligament is being sealed and cut with the LigaSure. B. Isolation and ligation of the ovarian ligament. In those patients who will be preserving the ovaries, the ovarian ligament is isolated and ligated. The IP ligament continues to provide blood supply to the ovaries.

dissection performed with the laparoscope is to have the assistant apply traction with countertraction to assist with the dissection.

The peritoneum next to the infundibulopelvic (IP) ligament overlying the pelvic sidewall is then opened either by incising it with the ABC or using the monopolar scissors. Once the ureter is visualized, the peritoneum above it can be opened further. A peritoneal window below the IP ligament but above the ureter can be bluntly opened with opposite traction by instruments both caudally and cephalad. The IP ligament is now isolated and separate from the ureter. Often with oncology cases, the ovaries will also be removed and the IP ligament can be ligated with the LigaSure or an endoscopic stapler. If the ovaries are to be preserved, then the utero-ovarian ligament is ligated instead of the IP ligament in the same fashion (Figure 2-7).

The dissection of the peritoneum toward the bladder and subsequent mobilization of the bladder can be performed with the ABC or monopolar scissors. With the uterus pushed in and upward, an incision is made in the vesicouterine peritoneum on the anterior aspect of the uterus using either the ABC or a monopolar device to create the bladder flap. The bladder pillars are divided and now the bladder is mobilized downward and dissected off the cervix.

Attention is now turned to identifying and exposing the uterine vessels laparoscopically. The broad ligament peritoneum is skeletonized to expose the vessels using the ABC. The uterine vessels should be identified in relation to the ureter. The uterine artery is then ligated alongside the uterus which differs from a radical hysterectomy where the uterine artery is ligated at the site of origin from the hypogastric artery. Once the uterine vessels are isolated, there are many options for ligation including cautery, suture ligation or laparoscopic clips.

The uterus can be anteflexed and the rectum pushed inferiorly so that the uterosacral ligaments are exposed. The uterosacral ligaments are then ligated using the LigaSure or other cautery and cut device or an endoscopic stapling device. Remember to keep the rectum and ureters visualized to avoid injury. As described by other authors, the harmonic ACE can be used to perform most of the steps for a TLH or total laparoscopic radical hysterectomy.[8]

A uterine manipulator ring within the vagina can be used and gently pushed inward to allow for the delineation of the area of the vagina to be incised both anteriorly and posteriorly. A blunt non-conducting vaginal probe can also be used and it is inserted into the vagina so that the vaginal-cervical junction can be delineated.[9] The anterior colpotomy is now performed with the anterior vaginal fornix on traction with the vaginal probe (Figure 2-8). The upper anterior vagina is then incised and the incision extended circumferentially to the posterior. The incision can be made with the ABC. Once this anterior and posterior colpotomy is complete, the uterus can be removed through the vagina. A single toothed tenaculum is placed through the colpotomy and is used to grasp and remove the specimen through the vagina. Once the uterus is removed, the pneumoperitoneum needs to be reestablished. This can be achieved by placing an appropriate instrument into the vagina or by placing a moist lap pad in the vagina. The vaginal edges are then closed with sutures laparoscopically. This can be approached in different ways. One technique is to use the EndoStitch and to place sutures in a running locked fashion (Figure 2-9). Interrupted sutures can also be placed and tied either intra- or extracorporally. The vaginal cuff is inspected for hemostasis. The pelvis is irrigated with saline to assess for bleeding.

Once the procedure had been completed, the trocars can be removed and the port sites closed. The fascia of all ports larger than 5-mm as well as the 5-mm ports that have been manipulated during the surgery should be closed with sutures.

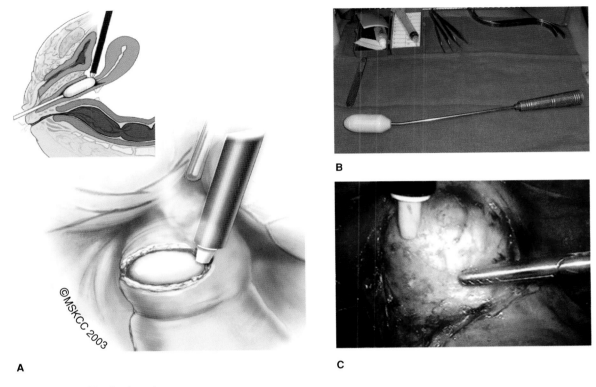

A

B

C

Figure 2-8 ▪ Vaginal probe.
A. Schematic representation of placement of the vaginal probe and subsequent anterior colpotomy. (Reproduced with permission from Medical Graphics, Memorial Sloan-Kettering Cancer Center.) B. One type of nonconducting vaginal probe. C. Vaginal probe inserted and delineating area to begin incision for colpotomy with the ABC.

PRE– AND POSTOPERATIVE MANAGEMENT

The preoperative management for those patients undergoing laparoscopy does not differ from those who undergo an open procedure. Bowel preparations prior to a major laparoscopic procedure can be useful since it may facilitate keeping the bowels retracted and away from the surgical field. The patient is instructed to only ingest clear liquids as well as to drink one bottle of fleet phospho-soda the day before the surgery. However, preoperative bowel preparation is an option and some gynecologic oncologists choose not to have their patients undergo a bowel prep.

The postoperative management differs after laparoscopy since the patients have often have less postoperative pain and require less narcotics.[10]

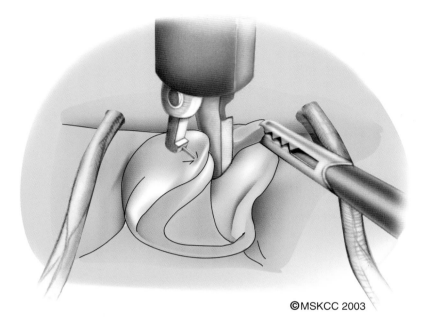

©MSKCC 2003

Figure 2-9 ▪ Closure of the vaginal cuff with the endostitch.
(Reproduced with permission from Medical Graphics, Memorial Sloan-Kettering Cancer Center.)

Patients are therefore able to ambulate more quickly. Intraoperative bowel manipulation is minimal with laparoscopy and patients are less likely to have a postoperative ileus. Patients are encouraged to resume a regular diet as early as postoperative day 1. In general, patients are sent home from the hospital sooner and are able to return to normal activities within a shorter time period.

COMPLICATIONS

Significant complications, some of which are specific to laparoscopy only, can be encountered during advanced complex laparoscopic procedures. Complications that can be encountered in any type of hysterectomy include major vascular injury and bleeding as well as injury to the intestines, ureters, or bladder. Understanding the types of complications associated with laparoscopy is important when incorporating the technique into practice.

Major vessel injury is rare. The open technique helps to minimize the risk of major vessel injury as it avoids the blind insertion of the Veress needle. Initially, with placement of the trocars, the deep inferior epigastric vessels can be injured and cause bleeding. This bleeding can be stopped by suturing the abdominal wall intraperitoneally with laparoscopic visualization.

Intestinal injury is not decreased with the use of the open technique. However, the location of the initial trocar placement in a patient with prior surgery may need to be adjusted to avoid bowel injury.

Before the procedure begins, it is crucial to identify the ureter and to trace its route from above the pelvic brim to the bladder. While injury to the ureters is reportedly minimal, the risk is much less if careful identification is performed prior to the resection. Small bladder injuries can be treated with continuous drainage with a foley whereas larger defects need to be repaired. Bladder injuries that are noted to be at the dome of the bladder or above the trigone can be closed primarily laparoscopically with sutures or with an endo-stitch.

Nerve injuries can occur if the patient is not properly positioned. However, the more common injuries are to the obturator and genitofemoral nerve which can also be injured at the time of laparotomy. Again, it is important to identify these structures laparoscopically before proceeding with the dissection.

The vaginal cuff is closed with laparoscopic sutures at the end of the TLH. An extremely rare complication is the breakdown of this repair and subsequent vaginal vault eviscerations. Technical problems or difficulty related to the closure may contribute to this complication. The management of this complication is surgical intervention. If there is intestinal prolapse, an abdominal exploratory procedure, either open or laparoscopically, is recommended to assess for bowel damage or ischemia.

Trocar (port) site incisional hernia is a complication unique to the technique of laparoscopy. This complication was first described by Fear in 1968 when he used laparoscopy for gynecologic diagnosis.[11] This complication is described within the surgical literature. Tonouchi et al. classify three types of trocar site hernias: early-onset type, late-onset type, and special type with dehiscence of whole abdominal wall. The overall true incidence of trocar site hernias is not known and has been more described relating to specific laparoscopic procedures.[12] Nezhat described a 0.2% risk of incisional hernia at the port site in a large series of 5300 women undergoing all types of laparoscopic gynecologic procedures.[13] In this series, hernias comprised omentum in seven cases and bowel in four cases and were seen in both 10-mm and 5-mm trocar sites.

Factors that may increase the risk of trocar site hernias include extensive manipulation of the port, stretching of the fascia to remove specimens, and not closing the fascial defect. All defects greater than 10-mm should be closed. The 5-mm port sites are not routinely closed; however, if the site was significantly manipulated or extended during the case, then it should be sutured closed.

Another complication associated with laparoscopy is the risk of trocar site metastasis or recurrence. Cases of recurrence at the laparotomy incision have also been reported. Therefore, this risk of surgical incisional recurrence is not unique to laparoscopy. The concern is that laparoscopy may lead to an increased risk of port site recurrence based on theoretical causes which include diffuse spread of tumor cells with pneumoperitoneum or direct implantation or contamination with retrieval of the specimen.[14] There is no data to support whether the development of port site metastasis is because of the surgical risk factors or because of the biology of the disease.

There have been cases described in the literature and the overall incidence reported varies.[15,16] In a large review of patients undergoing diagnostic laparoscopy or laparotomy for upper gastrointestinal malignancies, Shoup et al. reported a 0.79% rate of port site recurrences in the laparoscopy group versus a 0.86% rate of open incision site recurrences.[17] Abu-Rustum et al. reported a 0.97% rate of subcutaneous tumor implantation with laparoscopy for gynecologic malignancies. In this series, all the cases of recurrences were associated with carcinomatosis. There were no isolated port site recurrences identified.[18] It does appear that those patients with advanced disease with carcinomatosis and ascites at the time of laparoscopy may be at greater risk of developing a trocar site recurrence and therefore, patient selection is important.

The overall impact of this finding on survival is not known at this time. In order to help decrease this risk, all specimens should be minimally manipulated and removed through a laparoscopic bag.

OUTCOMES

Laparoscopy has a role in the treatment of ovarian, cervical and endometrial cancers. In general, laparoscopy has been shown to reduce postoperative pain and shorten hospital stay, leading to an earlier return to activities.[19] This can be translated into earlier initiation of adjuvant treatment for the gynecologic oncology patient.

TLH may be used for a number of gynecologic oncology indications but its role in oncology is most often reported for early stage endometrial cancer. There is data emerging that define the rate of recurrence and oncologic outcome for those undergoing laparoscopic procedures for oncologic reasons, particularly for endometrial cancer. Obermair et al. compared results of 510 patients undergoing either a TAH or TLH for primary surgical treatment of endometrial cancer.[20] They reported a 4.8% conversion rate to laparotomy for adhesions or to control bleeding. The recurrence rate was 4.0% in the laparoscopy group and 14.9% in the laparotomy group. The recurrence patterns were similar in the two groups and there were no cases of port site recurrences. Recently, the Gynecologic Oncology Group completed a trial which compared laparoscopic with abdominal surgery for endometrial cancer (GOG LAP-2 trial); we await the long-term results.

A significant change in treatment of endometrial cancer has occurred over the last few years leading to a less invasive surgical approach with a decrease in the use of whole pelvic radiation. Barakat et al. reviewed the outcomes of patients treated at Memorial Sloan-Kettering Cancer Center over a 12-year period. During this time, there was a shift towards more minimally invasive surgical treatment with an increase in incorporation of complete surgical staging for patients when feasible. With more completely staged patients, there was an associated decrease in the use of whole pelvic radiation adjuvant treatment. The important outcome was that there was no significant difference in survival between the two periods representing the different treatment modalities.[21]

TLH has minimal operative morbidity with decreased postoperative wound complications. The procedure is associated with a shorter and easier recovery period compared to conventional laparotomy. TLH does not appear to have a negative impact on long-term outcomes, however, data is still emerging. The basic steps of this procedure remain constant but the technique can be slightly altered. With appropriate training, TLH can be performed safely since a learning curve does exist for improving laparoscopic skills.[22] TLH is a feasible procedure that can and should be incorporated into the types of procedures performed at a single institution and offered to appropriate patients.[23]

REFERENCES

1. Childers JM, Surwit EA. Combined laparoscopic and vaginal surgery for the management of two cases of stage 1 endometrial cancer. *Gynecol Oncol*. 1992;45:46–51.

2. Reich H, DeCaprio J, McGlynn F. Laparoscopic hysterectomy. *J Gynecol Surg.* 1989;5:213–216.

3. Obermair A, Manolitsas TP, Leung Y, et al. Total laparoscopic hysterectomy versus total abdominal hysterectomy for obese women with endometrial cancer. *Int J Gynecol Cancer.* 2005;15:319–324.

4. Eltabbakh GH, Shamonki MI, Moody JM, et al. Hysterectomy for obese women with endometrial cancer: Laparoscopy or laparotomy? *Gynecol Oncol.* 2000;78:329–335.

5. Yu CK, Cutner A, Mould T, et al. Total laparoscopic hysterectomy as a primary surgical treatment for endometrial cancer in morbidly obese women. *BLOG.* 2005;112:115–117.

6. O'Hanlan KA, Dibble SL, Fisher DT. Total laparoscopic hysterectomy for uterine pathology: Impact of body mass index on outcomes. *Gynecol Oncol.* 2006;103: 938–941.

7. Elkington NM, Chou D. A review of total laparoscopic hysterectomy: Role, techniques and complications. *Curr Opin Obstet Gynecol.* 2006;18:380–384.

8. Frumovitz M, Ramirez PT. Total laparoscopic radical hysterectomy: Surgical technique and instrumentation. *Gynecol Oncol.* 2007;104:S13–S16.

9. McCartney AS, Johnson N. Using a vaginal tube to separate the uterus from the vagina during laparoscopic hysterectomy. *Obstet Gynecol.* 1995;85:293–296.

10. Eltabbakh GH. Analysis of survival after laparoscopy in women with endometrial cancer. *Cancer.* 2002;95:1894–1901.

11. Fear RE. Laparoscopy: A valuable aid in gynecologic diagnosis. *Obstet Gynecol.* 1968;31:297–309.

12. Tonouchi H, Ohmori Y, Kobayashi M, et al. Trocar site hernia. *Arch Surg.* 2004; 139:1248–1256.

13. Nezhat C, Nezhat F, Seidman DS, et al. Incisional hernias after operative laparoscopy. *J Laparoendosc Adv Surg Tech A.* 1997;7:111–115.

14. Wang PH, Yen MS, Yuan CC, et al. Port Site Metastasis after Laparoscopic-Assisted Vaginal Hyssterectomy for Endometrial Cancer: Possible Mechanisms and Prevention. *Gynecol Oncol.* 1997;66:151–155.

15. Huang KG, Wanf CJ, Chang TC, et al. Management of port-site metastasis after laparoscopic surgery for ovarian cancer. *Am J Obstet GYnecol.* 2003;189:16–21.

16. Ramirez PT, Frumovitz M, Wolf JK, Levenback C. Laparoscopic port-site metastasis in patients with gynecologic malignancies. *Int J Gynecol Cancer.* 2004;14:1070–1077.

17. Shoup M, Brennan MF, Karpeh, et al. Port site metastasis after diagnostic laparoscopy for upper gastrointestinal tract malignancies: An uncommon entity. *Ann Surg Oncol.* 2002;9:635–636.

18. Abu-Rustum NR, Rhee EH, Chi DS, et al. Subcutaneous tumor implantation after laparoscopic procedures in women with malignant disease. *Obstet Gynecol.* 2004;103:480–487.

19. Gemignani ML, Curtin JP, Zelmanovish J, et al. Laparoscopic-assisted vaginal hysterectomy for endometrial cancer: clinical outcomes and hospital charges. *Gynecol Oncol.* 1999;73:5–11.

20. Obermair A, Manolitsas TP, Leung Y, Hammond IG, and McCartney AJ. Total laparoscopic hysterectomy for endometrial cancer: Patterns of recurrence and survival. *Gynecologic Oncology* 2004;92:789–793.

21. Barakat RB, Lev G, Hummer AJ, Sonoda Y, Chi DS, Alektiar KM, et al. Twelve-year experience in the management of endometrial cancer: A change in surgical and postoperative radiation approaches. *Gynecol Oncol.* 2007;105:150–156.

22. Wattiez A, Soriano D, Cohen SB, et al. The learning curve of total laparoscopic hysterectomy: Comparative analysis of 1647 cases. *J Am Assoc Gynecol Laparosc.* 2002;9:339–345.

23. Garrett AJ, Nascimento MC, Nicklin JL, Perrin LC, Obermair A. Total laparoscopic hysterctomy: The Brisbane learning curve. *Aust N Z J Obstet Gynaecol.* 2007;47:65–69.

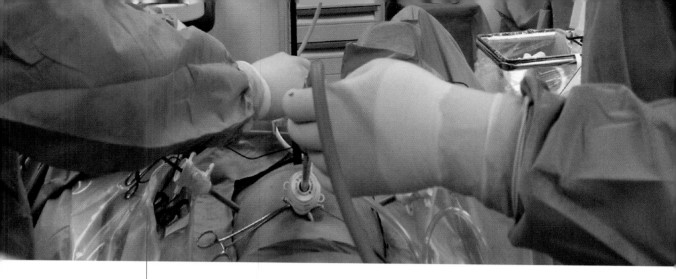

3 THE LAPAROSCOPIC RADICAL HYSTERECTOMY

Pedro T. Ramirez and Kathleen M. Schmeler

INTRODUCTION

Total laparoscopic radical hysterectomy for cervical cancer was described initially by Canis et al.[1] and Nezhat et al.[2] Since those initial reports, a number of other groups have published their experiences showing the feasibility and safety of this procedure for cervical cancer. The enthusiasm for this minimally invasive approach is because of several factors. Extensive literature supports the safety and oncologic efficacy of the procedure. Numerous studies have shown that recurrence and overall survival rates are equivalent in patients with early-stage cervical cancer who undergo radical hysterectomy by laparoscopy and laparotomy.[3–13]

Another key reason for the increasing popularity of the laparoscopic approach is the increasing level of proficiency by surgeons performing this procedure. Not only is there greater emphasis in training programs to assure that graduates are adequately trained to perform advanced laparoscopic surgery, but also there are plentiful opportunities for surgeons to attend training sessions through gynecologic oncology societies and industry-sponsored programs. This has significantly impacted on the learning curve of many physicians. In addition, the availability of much better equipment has added another level of safety to the laparoscopic approach. The increasing popularity of laparoscopic radical hysterectomy for early-stage cervical cancer is also because of the patient preference; this minimally invasive approach improves quality of life with its reduced perioperative morbidity and faster recovery time. This chapter will discuss the topics relevant to total laparoscopic radical hysterectomy as it pertains to patient selection, surgical technique, and overall outcomes.

INDICATIONS

The ideal patient for a total laparoscopic radical hysterectomy for cervical cancer has stage IA2 or IB1 disease. Occasionally, patients with stage IA1 disease at high risk for lymph node spread, such as those with extensive lymphovascular space invasion, high-grade disease, or high-risk histologic subtype (adenosquamous carcinoma, clear cell carcinoma, or neuroendocrine carcinoma) will also require radical hysterectomy and be considered candidates for laparoscopic surgery. In addition, carefully selected patients with stage IB2 or IIA disease have been included in studies of laparoscopic radical hysterectomy with good outcomes.

CONTRAINDICATIONS

Tumor factors

Similar to the open approach, cervical tumor size exceeding 4 cm in largest diameter remains a contraindication to laparoscopic radical hysterectomy. There are a number of reasons for this recommendation. First, patients with tumors larger than 4 cm have a higher risk of requiring postoperative radiotherapy to treat nodal metastases or cervical stromal invasion. Second, it may be more difficult to place a uterine manipulator around a larger lesion, thus limiting mobility of the uterus during the radical hysterectomy. Third, a larger tumor may interfere with the surgeon's ability to perform an adequate circumferential colpotomy to assure a 2-cm upper vaginal margin.

Other contraindications include the evidence of peritoneal carcinomatosis or distant metastatic disease. In addition, if the patient has evidence of grossly involved lymph nodes and these are documented to contain metastatic disease, there is no role for a radical hysterectomy.

Patient factors

Although there is no absolute weight restriction for laparoscopic radical hysterectomy, increasing body mass index (BMI) may increase rates of complications and conversion to laparotomy. Obese patients may also have a higher risk of anesthesia complications or difficulty with ventilation resulting from prolonged periods in the steep Trendelenburg position used for laparoscopic hysterectomy. In counseling patients with a large body habitus, it is important to emphasize that in the event that the anesthesiologist considers it unsafe to proceed with the laparoscopic approach, a laparotomy will be performed to complete the procedure. Obesity is thus not an absolute contraindication to laparoscopy but may be a determining factor for conversion based on the intraoperative physiologic and respiratory status of the patient.

Other factors that may exclude a patient from having a laparoscopic radical hysterectomy include multiple medical comorbidities such as severe cardiopulmonary disease and a history of multiple prior laparotomies, especially those performed for bowel resection, severe adhesions, ruptured appendix, or diverticular disease. Patients who are unable to be placed in a dorsal lithotomy position for a prolonged period because of their knee or hip problems also are not candidates for the laparoscopic approach.

Surgeon qualifications

The procedure should be offered to patients exclusively by surgeons who have achieved an excellent comfort level with laparoscopic simple hysterectomy and pelvic lymphadenectomy. An assistant surgeon who is also trained in advanced laparoscopic surgery is another requirement. The operating room team assisting in the case must also be familiar with the steps of the procedure and the instrumentation routinely used during total laparoscopic radical hysterectomy.

PREOPERATIVE EVALUATION

The preoperative evaluation should include confirmation of the histologic diagnosis followed by a thorough pelvic examination to document that the disease is limited to the cervix. A chest x-ray is performed to assure that there is no evidence of disease spread to the lungs. Although not absolutely required, computed tomography of the abdomen and pelvis is often performed to detect any evidence of disease spread. If there is evidence of spread to the lymph nodes or intraperitoneal cavity, then the patient can be spared unnecessary general anesthesia and surgery.

Patients should be counseled regarding the options of laparotomy and laparoscopy as the approaches for radical hysterectomy. Patients having the laparoscopic approach can anticipate a faster recovery with earlier resumption of daily activities, reduced requirements for pain medication, faster return of bowel function, and earlier discharge from the hospital than with the open approach. In addition, total blood loss and transfusion rates are lower with the laparoscopic approach. However, the intraoperative time is usually higher, particularly during the initial learning phase of the surgeon. It should be emphasized that preliminary retrospective data shows that oncologic outcomes are equivalent with the laparoscopic and the open approach.

SURGICAL TECHNIQUE

Patient preparation and positioning

The day prior to surgery, the patient is placed on a clear liquid diet and undergoes a mechanical bowel preparation. Prior to the induction of anesthesia, elastic stockings and external pneumatic compression devices are placed on the lower extremities to prevent thromboembolic disease. The use of unfractionated heparin or low-molecular-weight heparin can also be considered.

After induction of general anesthesia, the patient is placed in the low lithotomy position using Allen stirrups. Typically, the patient's arms are tucked at her sides. The patient is then placed in the steep Trendelenburg position.

Insertion of trocars

A 12-mm trocar is placed at the level of the umbilicus and introduced into the abdominal cavity under direct visualization. In patients with a prior midline incision, the initial entry into the abdominal cavity is made approximately 2 cm below the left costal margin at the level of the midclavicular line to avoid injury to bowel adherent to the anterior abdominal wall.

Once the first trocar has been safely introduced into the abdominal cavity, the cavity is insufflated. The intra-abdominal pressure is maintained at 16 mm Hg.

Two additional 12-mm trocars are then placed in the right and left lower quadrants, and an additional 5-mm trocar is inserted in the midline above the pubic symphysis.

Entry into the retroperitoneal space

The pelvis and abdomen are thoroughly explored to rule out intraperitoneal disease. The round ligaments are transected bilaterally. An incision is made in the peritoneum over the psoas muscle immediately lateral to the infundibulopelvic ligament. The infundibulopelvic ligament is retracted medially to permit identification of the ureter. The iliac vessels are also exposed at this time. The lymph-bearing tissue along the pelvis is then evaluated for obvious metastatic disease. Any suspicious pelvic lymph nodes are removed and sent for frozen-section examination. If these are positive for metastatic disease, the radical hysterectomy is aborted and a para-aortic lymph node dissection is performed to determine the field of radiation.

Opening of the pararectal and paravesical spaces

The paravesical space is opened by placing medial traction of the obliterated umbilical artery and dissecting on the loose aerolar tissue lateral to the vessel. The space is opened until the pelvic floor is visualized. The space medial to the obliterated umbilical artery is also dissected and exposed. The pararectal space is opened by dissecting the area between the ureter and the internal iliac artery, posterior to the uterine vessels.

Identification and transection of the uterine artery

After the pararectal and paravesical spaces are completely opened, the uterine artery and vein are identified and transected at the point of origin from the internal iliac vessels. The uterine vessels are transected together rather than separately.

Mobilization of the bladder

The visceral peritoneum overlying the interface between the bladder and uterus is incised and dissected free of the cervix. We take particular care at this point in the procedure to completely separate the bladder fibers from the anterior vagina as this allows for adequate resection for a 2 cm upper vaginal margin, and it also facilitates closure of the vaginal cuff at the end of the procedure.

Dissection of the parametrial tissue

The ureters are separated from their medial attachments to the peritoneum. The parametrial tissue is then brought over the ureters, and the ureters are dissected to the point of their insertion into the bladder bilaterally. The lateral aspect of the vesicouterine ligament is then divided, and the bladder is further mobilized inferiorly to ensure adequate vaginal margins.

Preoperative ureteral stent placement to assist with dissection and to prevent injury is controversial. The risks may outweigh the benefits, as stent placement can result in bleeding, edema, or damage to the ureter. In addition, it may predispose the ureter to injury caused by immobility.

Division of the uterosacral ligaments

The uterus is anteflexed, and the peritoneum overlying the interface between the rectum and posterior vagina is then incised, exposing the rectovaginal space. The attachments between the rectum and the vagina are cut in the midline, exposing the uterosacral ligaments, which are then transected.

Removal of the specimen

The cervix and uterus are now free of all their vascular and suspensory attachments and can be removed. The specimen, including the upper vaginal margin, cervix, and uterus, is completely separated from the upper vagina and removed while attached to a modified vaginal ring and uterine manipulator developed at the University of Texas M.D. Anderson Cancer Center.[14] The vaginal cuff is sutured laparoscopically.

POSTOPERATIVE MANAGEMENT

In the immediate postoperative period, patients generally receive intravenous pain medication as needed supplemented with oral analgesics. All patients are transitioned to oral analgesics as they demonstrate tolerating their diet. Patients consume a clear liquid diet the evening of the surgery and a regular diet the morning after surgery. All patients have a Foley catheter placed at the time of surgery, and this is not removed until 7 to 10 days postoperatively. Patients are prepared for discharge from the hospital on postoperative day 1. Patients are taught how to care for their bladder catheter and discharged home with oral antibiotics for prophylaxis while the catheter is in place. A voiding trial is scheduled 7 to 10 days postoperatively. An alternative to placing a Foley catheter is to teach patients self-catheterization prior to discharge while hospitalized.

Patients are re-evaluated 4 to 6 weeks after their surgery. Subsequent follow-up includes a routine pelvic examination with a Pap smear every 3 months for 2 years and then every 6 months for the next 3 years.

COMPLICATIONS

The intraoperative complications in patients undergoing laparoscopic radical hysterectomy include those typical of routine laparoscopic gynecologic surgery: injury to the bowel, bladder, blood vessels, or ureter. Vascular injury is the most common and may occur during initial trocar placement, lymph node dissection, or dissection of the parametrial tissue. Venous injuries are typically controlled with simple pressure or hemostatic agents. Arterial injuries are usually more challenging to address and often require placement of hemoclips or suturing.

Patients may also experience neuropathy following extensive pelvic lymphadenectomy. The genitofemoral nerve may be injured during removal of the external iliac lymph nodes, resulting in parasthesia of the ipsilateral mons, labia majorum, and skin overlying the femoral triangle. Obturator neuropathy may also occur, resulting in sensory loss of the upper medial thigh and motor weakness in the hip adductors. If complete transection of the obturator nerve occurs, immediate repair using microsurgical technique should be performed. Fortunately, most neurologic injuries are usually transient and resolve with minimal intervention.

OUTCOMES

More than 400 patients have been reported to have undergone total laparoscopic radical hysterectomy. Although no randomized trials have

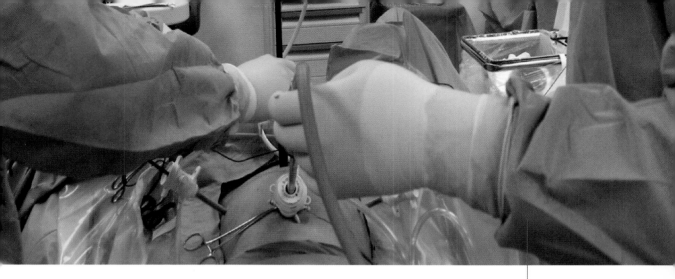

TECHNIQUE OF LAPAROSCOPIC TRANSPERITONEAL PELVIC LYMPHADENECTOMY

4

Eric Leblanc, Fabrice Narducci, Jerome Phalippou,
Eric Lambaudie, Malik Boukerrou, and Denis Querleu

The accuracy of current imaging methods for retroperitoneal node status assessment is not satisfactory. Morphologic imaging techniques (CT scan and MRI) have a sensitivity of less than 80%[1] although a significant improvement is awaited from the use of ultrasmall superparamagnetic iron oxide (USPIO) with MRI.[2] Functional imaging such as PET/CT scan does not seem to be superior to CT scan or MRI.[3] Given that the size of metastasis is the limiting factor for detection, node retrieval remains the best means to evaluate the true status of lymph nodes.[4] Pelvic lymph node dissection remains a key part of the staging procedures of most epithelial invasive gynecologic pelvic tumors.

Historically, D. Dargent[5] was the first to perform pelvic lymph nodes dissection laparoscopy. He advocated a bilateral extraperitoneal approach, that he referred to as the retroperitoneal panoramic pelviscopy. This approach is complex to perform, with a significant morbidity and not very adaptable if a concurrent intra-abdominal operative step is required. The transperitoneal approach initially promoted by D. Querleu[6] is the preferred approach to perform pelvic lymph node dissections in gynecologic cancer patients. Its indications, technique, and results are described in this chapter.

DEFINITIONS

The distribution of a pelvic node dissection is the interiliac area, located between the internal and external iliac vessels. Its boundaries are the common iliac bifurcation cranially, the iliopubic branch with the Cooper's ligament and the obturator foramen caudally, the psoas muscle laterally, the superior vesical artery medially, the peritoneum covering these structures superficially, and the obturator nerve deeply. A systematic pelvic lymphadenectomy removes all nodes located in this field, including lateral to the external iliac artery, between artery and vein and between external iliac vein and the obturator nerve as well as nodes around the internal iliac vessels down to the obturator nerve.

INDICATIONS

Ovarian cancer

Since nodal involvement is frequent and ubiquitous even in apparently localized ovarian carcinoma, a bilateral pelvic lymphadenectomy is to be considered part of the staging of any invasive epithelial adnexal tumor along with the infrarenal para-aortic dissection and comprehensive peritoneal staging.[7,8] This staging is feasible through laparoscopy[9] and indicated for early tumors in all subtypes and substages except in stage IA grade I mucinous carcinomas.[10] Although the survival effect is controversial,[11,12] the result of the exploration impacts on further management. In more advanced cases, the indication of a systematic lymphadenectomy is more controversial. If a survival benefit has been shown in the case of a bulky disease,[13] this advantage is not so clear in normal size nodes, especially after chemotherapy.

the node, the higher the risk of rupture. Thus, in our opinion, 3 cm is the limit in size for a safe laparoscopic dissection.

ADVANTAGES AND COMPLICATIONS OF LAPAROSCOPIC PELVIC LYMPHADENECTOMIES

Advantages

Besides the esthetic advantage of a minimal scarring, laparoscopy can provide fewer adhesions than laparotomy[26,27] which is beneficial especially if postoperative pelvic irradiation may be indicated. A quicker postoperative recovery offers a reduced length of stay after the use of laparoscopy.[28,29]

In spite of a longer operative time than laparotomy,[29] laparoscopic lymphadenectomy is a safe procedure. Complications described above are rare in large series (Table 4-1). So far, two deaths have been reported in the gynecologic literature (one related to the initial trocar insertion in a common iliac vein, the other to a pulmonary embolism after a laparotomy indicated to fix a bowel herniation through a trocar site incision). They both happened in a team who had limited laparoscopic experience.[30]

Complications

Hemorrhage

Bleeding is not rare during this procedure. Most bleeding is minimal and represents normal lymphohematic oozing; its amount can be reduced by a systematic dissection avoiding any morcellation of nodal groups. Localized bleeders are first controlled by packing, using the surrounding tissues or a guaze or sponge. After packing the area for a while, the field is cleared with saline irrigation and the pressure is released. Generally bleeding will stop or will be reduced enough to enable the surgeon to fix it using bipolar coagulation or clips. If bleeding remains significant, or in the case of a large iliac vessel injury, a laparotomy must be quickly carried out. Clips or endoscopic clamps should not be applied without a clear visibility, at the risk of increasing the vascular damage.

Pre- and intraoperative knowledge of the anatomy[31] as well as the knowledge of some commonly injured areas are important. Care must be paid when dissecting the anterior obturator fossa because of the anterior obturator vessels that may be present,[32] the deep lumbo-sciatic fossa dissection with several branches from the hypogastric pedicle is difficult to clear, and laterally the presence of vessels extending from the psoas muscle

Table 4–1 **COMPLICATIONS OF LAPAROSCOPIC PELVIC LYMPHADENECTOMIES IN SOME LARGE SERIES**

	N	Indications	Age	BMI	Failures	Complications	Vascular Injuries	Injuries	Lymphatic
Leblanc 2007*	686	Cervix: 436 Endometrium: 150 Adnexa: 102	Av: 42.3 (9-83)	Av: 26 (15.4-61.8)	12 Adhesions: 2 Fixed node: 8 Obesity: 2	68 (10%) Perop: 2% Postop: 7.8%	10 (0 lap)	Ureter 3 (1 lap) Bladder 1 Bowel 1 (1 lap) Nerve 3	35 (8 legedemas)
Köhler 2005[41]	49†	Cervix: 343 Endometrium: 112 Ovary: 44	Av: 49 (14-85)	Av: 25.9 (15.4-49.7)	—	53 (8.7%) Perop: 2,9 Postop: 5,8	3 (2 lap)	Bowel: 3 Nerve: 16	3 lymphoceles, (6 legedemas)
Scribner 2001[30]	10‡	Endometrium: 95 Ovary: 8	Av: 66 (24-92)	Av: 30.8 (15.9-56.1)	30 Obesity: 12 Adhesions: 5 Carinomatosis: 5	11 (11%) Perop: 3% Postop: 8% (2 deaths)	1 lap and death	Bladder 1, ureter 1	—

* Updated from Querleu D, Leblance E, Cartron G, Narducci F, Ferron G, Martel P. Audit of preoperative and early complications of laparoscopic lymph node dissection in 1000 gynecologic cancer patients. *Am J Obstet Gynecol.* 2006;195(5):1287-1292.

† From a series of 650 pelvic and/or para-aortic lymphadenectomies.

‡ Pelvic and para-aortic lymphadenectomy.

to external iliac vessels, especially close to the common iliac bifurcation, may be a source of serious bleeding during the latero-iliac dissection. When compared to laparotomy, the rate of blood transfusion, is lower for laparoscopy.[23]

Pelvic nerve complications

The transsection of the obturator or the femorocutaneous nerves is a very rare event unless a node is fixed to the nerve; thermal injury during dissection is the usual cause of postoperative dysesthesia. The use of bipolar current should be preferred for tissue coagulation around nerves.

Urinary complications

Ureteral damage may be caused by the dissection of fixed nodes, or thermal injury. Bladder injury may occur during anterior dissection. Methylene blue test may be useful if a bladder injury is suspected. Intraoperative or postoperative stenting of suspicious ureters may prevent fistulas.

Bowel complications

These complications are infrequent. Perforations can be secondary to adhesiolysis. This step should be performed gently, using sharp dissection rather than monopolar current. An occult bowel perforation can occur as well if instruments are used outside the laparoscopic view. Any bowel perforation or suspicious area should be sutured either laparoscopically or directly through an enlarged trocar site. Secondary bowel obstructions were reported as a result of herniation through 10 mm and larger port sites, which should be closed at the completion of surgery.

Lymphatic complications

The main complication is lympatic leakage resulting in lymphatic ascites. Only symptomatic lymphocysts should be treated. Methods vary from imaging guided sclerotherapy or drainage[33] to the surgical marsupialization through laproscopy[34] to even laparotomy in the case of an abcess. Ascites is usually managed with drainage.

The most serious sequelae of pelvic lymphadenectomy (not specific to laparoscopy) is leg edema. It may occur after surgery alone but is more frequently observed when external beam radation therapy is combined with surgery.[35–37] Although difficult to predict, the risk seems low but the patient should be informed of this possibility.[38]

Port site metastases

Very few isolated port site implants are reported in the literature.[35] Morcellation of involved nodes along with their direct extraction (without bag) is likely to be the main reason of this complication.[20] Prognosis may be different when trocar site implants are associated with a peritoneal carcinomatosis.[39] Port site irrigation to prevent metastasis, is controversial.[40]

CONCLUSION

When compared to laparotomy, laparoscopy induces less complications, especially for high risk patients.[23] Most perioperative complications are correlated with the surgeon's level of experience.[41,42] Although variable,[43] the plateau of the learning curve (stable node yield and operative time) is usually achieved after 10 to 20 consecutive cases, as demonstrated experimentally,[44] and clinically.[41,45]

Laparoscopy is now a recognized method to perform pelvic lymphadenectomies which, in experienced hands, is comparable to laparotomy with regards to surgical outcomes.

REFERENCES

1. Scheidler J, Haricak H, Yu KK, Subak L, Segal MR. Radiological evaluation of lymph node metastases in patients with cervical cancer. A meta-analysis. *JAMA*. 1997;278(13):1096–1101.
2. Rockall AG, Sohaib SA, Harisinghani MG, et al. Diagnostic performance of nanoparticle-enhanced magnetic resonance imaging in the diagnosis of lymph node metastases in patients with endometrial and cervical cancer. *J Clin Oncol*. 2005; 23(12):2813–2821.
3. Havrilesky LJ, Kulasingam SL, Matchar DB, Myers ER. FDG-PET for management of cervical and ovarian cancer. *Gynecol Oncol*. 2005;97(1):183–191.
4. Sironi S, Buda A, Picchio M, et al. Lymph node metastasis in patients with clinical early-stage cervical cancer: Detection with integrated FDG PET/CT. *Radiology*. 2006;238(1):272–279.
5. Dargent D. *L'envahissement Ganglionnaire Pelvien*. McGraw Hill; 1986:137.
6. Querleu D, Leblanc E, Castelain B. Laparoscopic pelvic lymphadenectomy in the staging of early carcinoma of the cervix. *Am J Obstet Gynecol*. 1991;164(2):579–581.

7. Trimbos JB. Staging of early ovarian cancer and the impact of lymph node sampling. *Int J Gynecol Cancer*. 2000;10(S1):8–11.

8. Harter P, Gnauert K, Hils R, et al. Pattern and clinical predictors of lymph node metastases in epithelial ovarian cancer. *Int J Gynecol Cancer*. 2007;17(6):1238–1244.

9. Leblanc E, Sonoda Y, Narducci F, Ferron G, Querleu D. Laparoscopic staging of early ovarian carcinoma. *Curr Opin Obstet Gynecol*. 2006;18(4):407–412.

10. Morice P, Joulie F, Camatte S, et al. Lymph node involvement in epithelial ovarian cancer: Analysis of 276 pelvic and paraaortic lymphadenectomies and surgical implications. *J Am Coll Surg*. 2003;197(2):198–205.

11. Maggioni A, Benedetti Panici P, Dell, Anna T, et al. Randomised study of systematic lymphadenectomy in patients with epithelial ovarian cancer macroscopically confined to the pelvis. *Br J Cancer*. 2006;95(6):699–704.

12. Trimbos JB, Parmar M, Vergote I, et al. Impact of adjuvant chemotherapy and surgical staging in early-stage ovarian carcinoma: European Organisation for Research and Treatment of Cancer-Adjuvant ChemoTherapy in Ovarian Neoplasm trial. *J Natl Cancer Inst*. 2003;95(2):113–125.

13. Panici PB, Maggioni A, Hacker N, et al. Systematic aortic and pelvic lymphadenectomy versus resection of bulky nodes only in optimally debulked advanced ovarian cancer: A randomized clinical trial. *J Natl Cancer Inst*. 2005;97(8):560–566.

14. Kong A, Samera I, Collingwood M, Williams C, Kitchener H. Adjuvant radiotherapy for stage I endometrial cancer. *Cochrane Database Syst Rev*. 2007(2):CD003916.

15. Houvenaeghel G, Lelievve L, Rigouard Al, et al. Residual pelvic lymph node involvement after concomitant chemoradiation for locally advanced cervical cancer. *Gynecol Oncol*. 2006;102(1):74–79.

16. Abu-Rustum N, Barakat R. Observations on the role of circumflex iliac node resection and the etiology of lower extremity lymph edema following pelvic lymphadenectopmy for gynecologic malignancy. *Gynecol Oncol*. 2007;106(1):4–5.

17. Homesley HD, Burdy BN, Sedlis A, Adcock L. Radiation therapy versus pelvic node resection for carcinoma of the vulva with positive groin nodes. *Obstet Gynecol*. 1986;68(6):733–740.

18. Klemm P, Marnitz S, Kohler C, Braig U, Schneider A. Clinical implication of laparoscopic pelvic lymphadenectomy in patients with vulvar cancer and positive groin nodes. *Gynecol Oncol*. 2005;99(1):101–105.

19. Holub Z, Jabor A, Kliment L, Lukac J, Voracek J. Laparoscopic lymph node dissection using ultrasonically activated shears: Comparison with electrosurgery. *J Laparoendosc Adv Surg Tech A*. 2002;12(3):175–180.

20. Nezhat F, Yadav J, Rahaman J, Gretz H, Gardner GJ, Cohen CJ. Laparoscopic lymphadenectomy for gynecologic malignancies using ultrasonically activated shears: Analysis of first 100 cases. *Gynecol Oncol*. 2005;97(3):813–819.

21. Sert BM, Abeler VM. Robotic-assisted laparoscopic radical hysterectomy (Piver type III) with pelvic node dissection—Case report. *Eur J Gynaecol Oncol*. 2006;27(5):531–533.

22. Franchi M, Trimbos JB, Zanaboni F, et al. Randomized trial of drains versus no drains following radiacal hysterectomy and pelvic lymph node dissection:

A European Organisation for Research and Treatment of Cancer-Gynaecological Cancer Group (EORTC-GCG) study in 234 patients. *Eur J Cancer.* 2007;43(8): 1265–1268.

23. Scribner DR Jr, Walker JL, Johnson GA, McMeekin SD, Gold MA, Mannel RS. Surgical management of early-stage endometrial cancer in the elderly: Is laparoscopy feasible? *Gynecol Oncol.* 2001;83(3):563–568.

24. Scribner DR Jr, Walker JL, Johnson GA, McMeekin SD, Gold MA, Mannel RS. Laparoscopic pelvic and paraaortic lymph node dissection in the obese. *Gynecol Oncol.* 2002;84(3):426–430.

25. Eltabbakh GH, Shamonki MI, Moody JM, Garafano LL. Hysterectomy for obese women with endometrial cancer: Laparoscopy or laparotomy? *Gynecol Oncol.* 2000;78(3 Pt 1):329–335.

26. Fowler JM, Hartenbach EM, Reynolds HT, et al. Pelvic adhesion formation after pelvic lymphadenectomy: Comparison between transperitoneal laparoscopy and extraperitoneal laparotomy in a porcine model. *Gynecol Oncol.* 1994;55(1): 25–28.

27. Chen MD, Teigen GA, Reynolds HT, Johnson PR, Fowler JM. Laparoscopy versus laparotomy: An evaluation of adhesion formation after pelvic and paraaortic lymphadenectomy in a porcine model. *Am J Obstet Gynecol.* 1998;178(3):499–503.

28. Morelli M, Noia R, Costantino A, et al. Laparoscopic lymphadenectomy as treatment of endometrial cancer. *Minerva Ginecol.* 2007;59(2):111–116.

29. Panici PB, Plotti F, Zullo MA, et al. Pelvic lymphadenectomy for cervical carcinoma: Laparotomy extraperitoneal, transperitoneal or laparoscopic approach? A randomized study. *Gynecol Oncol.* 2006;103(3):859–864.

30. Scribner DR Jr, Walker JL, Johnson GA, McMeekin SD, Gold MA, Mannel RS. Laparoscopic pelvic and paraaortic lymph node dissection: Analysis of the first 100 cases. *Gynecol Oncol.* 2001;82(3):498–503.

31. Benedetti-Panici P, Maneschi F, Scambia G, Greggi S, Mancuso S. Anatomic abnormalities of the retroperitoneum during aortic and pelvic lymphadenectomy. *Am J Obstet Gynecol.* 1994;170(1pt1):111–116.

32. Lee YS. Early experience with laparoscopic pelvic lymphadenectomy in women with gynecologic malignancy. *J Am Assoc Gynecol Laparosc.* 1999;6(1):59–63.

33. Karcaaltincaba M, Akhan O. Radiologic imaging and percutaneous treatment of pelvic lymphocele. *Eur J Radiol.* 2005;55(3):340–354.

34. Recio FO, Ghamande S, Hempling RE, Piver MS. Effective management of pelvic lymphocysts by laparoscopic marsupialization. *JSLS.* 1999;3(2):97–102.

35. Kehoe SM, Abu-Rustum NR. Transperitoneal laparoscopic pelvic and paraaortic lymphadenectomy in gynecologic cancers. *Curr Treat Options Oncol.* 2006;7(2):93–101.

36. Matsuura Y, Kawage T, Toki N, Tanaka M, Kashimura M. Long-standing complications after treatment for cancer of the uterine cervix—Clinical significance of medical examination at 5 years after treatment. *Int J Gynecol Cancer.* 2006;16(1): 294–297.

37. Werngren-Elgström M, Lidman D. Lymphoedema of the lower extremities after surgery and radiation therapy of cancer of the cervix. *Scand J Plast reconstr Surg Hand Surg*. 1994;28(4):289–293.

38. Gary D. Lymphoedema diagnosis and management. *J Am Acad Nurse Pract*. 2007;19(2):72–78.

39. Wang PH, Yuan CC, Chao KC, Yen MS, Ng HT, Chao HT. Squamous cell carcinoma of the cervix after laparoscopic surgery. A case report. *J Reprod Med*. 1997;42(12):801–804.

40. Wittich P, Mearadji A, Marquet RL, Bonjer HJ. Irrigation of port sites: Prevention of port site metastases? *J Laparoendosc Adv Surg Tech A*. 2004;14(3):125–129.

41. Köhler C, Klemm P, Schau A, et al. Introduction of transperitoneal lymphadenectomy in a gynecologic oncology center: Analysis of 650 laparoscopic pelvic and/or paraaortic transperitoneal lymphadenectomies. *Gynecol Oncol*. 2004;95(1): 52–61.

42. Querleu D, Leblanc E, Carton G, Narducci F, Ferron G, Martel P. Audit of preoperative and early complications of laparoscopic lymph node dissection in 1000 gynecologic cancer patients. *Am J Obstet Gynecol*. 2006;195(5):1287–1292.

43. Altgassen C, Possover M, Krause N, Plaul K, Michels W, Schneider A. Establishing a new technique of laparoscopic pelvic and para-aortic lymphadenectomy. *Obstet Gynecol*. 2000;95(3):348–352.

44. Querleu D, Lanvin D, Elhage A, Henry-Buisson B, Leblanc E. An objective experimental assessment of the learning curve for laparoscopic surgery: The example of pelvic and para-aortic lymph node dissection. *Eur J Obstet Gynecol Reprod Biol*. 1998;81(1):55–58.

45. Fowler JM, Carter JR, Carlson JW, et al. Lymph node yield from laparoscopic lymphadenectomy in cervical cancer: A comparative study. *Gynecol Oncol*. 1993;51(2):187–192.

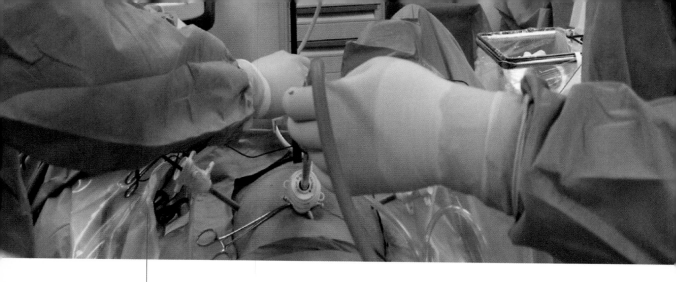

5

PARA–AORTIC LYMPH NODE DISSECTION THROUGH A TRANSPERITONEAL AND RETROPERITONEAL APPROACH

Denis Querleu and Eric Leblanc

With the development of laparoscopic infrarenal node dissections in the early 1990s,[1,2] the last frontiers of laparoscopic surgery in gynecologic oncology were reached—except for laparoscopic exenterations that still remain investigational. Like its open equivalent, laparoscopic aortic node dissection can be performed using transperitoneal or extraperitoneal techniques. Credit must be given to late Daniel Dargent and Joel Childers for their signification contributions to pioneering the technique.[3] This operation is not difficult for an experienced oncologic surgeon, and may be routinely carried out by laparoscopy. The proportion of patients in whom the operation can be satisfactorily completed by this new approach is well over 90% in the experience of the leading teams in this field.[4,5]

INDICATIONS

Indications for aortic dissection

Aortic node dissection is part of most gynecologic oncology procedures in primary or recurrent gynaecologic malignancies. It is standard for adnexal cancers. It is controversial in early endometrial cancers but routinely performed by the majority of gynaecologic oncologists in the case of positive pelvic nodes or in high-risk cases (stage ICG3, papillary serous subtypes). In early cervical carcinomas, some perform routine aortic dissection, while others perform aortic dissections only in patients with positive pelvic nodes. In advanced cervical cancers, the concept of surgical staging is not widely accepted, although this procedure may spare the node negative patient unnecessary para-aortic irradiation, and the node positive patient unnecessary primary surgery or exenteration for pelvic recurrence.

Indications and contraindications for laparoscopic aortic dissection

Indications for laparoscopic aortic node dissection includes situations where staging is the only goal of the operation, as in the case of advanced cervical cancers, or for the reassessment of apparently early but inadequately staged adnexal malignancies, or in the setting of workup before pelvic exenteration. Aortic dissection may also be part of the comprehensive surgical management of early gynaecologic malignancies.

When the surgical management of the primary disease requires an open approach to remove bulky disease, laparoscopic surgery has no role. When performing laparoscopic surgery for ovarian cancer it is crucial to avoid tumor rupture and/or contamination of the abdominal wall, which is possible only when the tumor size is less than 5 cm.

Indications for transperitoneal or extraperitoneal approach

Several parameters are considered. Feasibility is the first element of choice. When the technical conditions are not optimal, for instance in obese patients, it is advisable to try the extraperitoneal approach, first as it may be possible to overcome a failure of the extraperitoneal approach using the transperitoneal route, whereas the opposite is not possible. Additionally, the extraperitoneal route should be considered first choice when a history of laparotomy suggests the presence of extensive intraperitoneal adhesions.

The main benefits of the extraperitoneal approach are a reduction of postoperative de novo adhesions, as demonstrated in an experimental study,[5] less postsurgical pain and easy access to the left infrarenal area, no bowel loops in the way, especially in obese patients. As a consequence, the patients who may require extended field radiation may benefit from the retroperitoneal approach. This includes patients presenting with an advanced cervical cancer and patients with high-risk endometrial cancers.

Considering the better surgical pain attached to the choice of the extraperitoneal approach, we generally adopt the extraperitoneal route even when an transperitoneal procedure such as reassessment of adnexal malignancy or hysterectomy is required for the surgical management. In such cases, a "combined" approach is used. The first step is a diagnostic transperitoneal laparoscopy. A retroperitoneal aortic (and common iliac, and when required and possible pelvic) dissection is then performed. Finally, the transperitoneal view is re-established, the trocars used for the extraperitoneal approach are pushed into the peritoneal cavity, and the transperitoneal steps of the operation are carried out.

CONTRAINDICATIONS

There are a few definite contra-indications for laparoscopic aortic dissection. General contraindications for laparoscopy are standard. A history of laparotomy is not a contraindication, but in the setting of known severe adhesions an extraperitoneal approach should be attempted first. Practically, the main issues are oncologic. Patients who will not benefit from the pathologic staging—such as elderly patients who will not be suitable for extended field radiation therapy with concomitant chemotherapy or patients with distant metastasis identified at the time of positron emission tomography or patients with node metastasis identified at imaging and cytologically confirmed—do not benefit from laparoscopic staging.

Another issue to be considered is the safe removal of bulky nodes via the laparoscope. On one hand, surgical debulking of enlarged aortic nodes is an acceptable procedure but its benefit has never been demonstrated in a randomised study. Additionally, abdominal wall contamination, or spillage of cancer cells in the retroperitoneal space is a concern. Finally, the dissection of fixed nodes may harm large vessels, leading to emergency laparotomies for vascular repair. Our policy is to laparoscopically remove obviously diseased nodes up to 3 cm, which are generally cleavable from the large vessels, taking care not to break the node capsule by avoiding grasping and using gentle and cautious blunt dissection and retrieving the nodes via an endoscopic bag.

SETUP, PATIENT POSITIONING, AND EQUIPMENT

The patient gives informed consent to the laparoscopic procedure and is ready for a laparotomy in case of technical difficulty or complication. The operation is performed under general anesthesia. As the patient set up is different for the extraperitoneal and transperitoneal approach, it will be described separately.

For the transperitoneal surgery, the patient is placed in the supine position without any flexion of the hips, as the flexed legs may limit the movements of the instruments in all the directions of the abdomen. The legs are placed in a 30-degree angle so that the surgeon may stand between them when exploring the upper quadrants of the abdomen. It is advisable to use a monitor screen placed at the head of the patient. For the extraperitoneal surgery, the patient lays flat on the operating table. The senior surgeon stands on the left side of the patient and the assistant stands on surgeon's left side; both watch a monitor screen placed on the right side of the patient.

The operative procedure requires 4.5-mm scissors, grasping forceps, irrigation-aspiration device, and bipolar coagulation forceps. We advise bipolar forceps with flat tips for fine hemostasis close to the ureter, the bowel, or large vessels. Endoscopic clips must be available to control bleeding from large vessels or to radiologically localize fixed nodes. We routinely use sponges to clean the operative field and facilitate suction. More sophisticated instruments such as argon beam coagulator, ultrasonic dissectors, or thermal fusion devices can be used at surgeon's choice but do not add to the safety and duration of the procedure. In a pilot study (not yet published), we found that systematic lymphostasis using the ultrasonic dissector (Ultracision®) reduced the lymphocyst formation rate after extraperitoneal dissection.

General principles must be recalled: the surgeon must be trained in aortic dissection, management of large vessel injury, and laparoscopic surgery. It has been shown that 15 cases under supervision are required to train a fellow.[6] In addition, the surgeon must be aware of the numerous anatomical variants of the arteries and veins of the area, including ectopic renal arteries and double vena cava.[7]

PRE- AND POSTOPERATIVE MANAGEMENT

Pre- and postoperative management are standard. Cefazolin is used in our institution for antibioprophylaxis. Prevention of venous thrombosis is essential; we use low dose of low-molecular-weight heparin. Positioning of the patient must avoid any compression of the legs. Postoperatively the diet is advanced as soon as possible and the patient is generally discharged on the first postoperative day.

TECHNIQUE

Transperitoneal para-aortic lymphadenectomy

A pneumoperitoneum is created. We routinely use a left upper quadrant approach for the Veress needle. A 10-mm laparoscope is introduced through an umbilical incision in patients without history of laparotomy. In case of the previous laparotomy, a syringe test is routinely performed in order to choose the safest location, usually above the umbilicus. As an additional precaution, the direct vision technique with the Endotip trocar is used for the introduction of the 10-mm trocar. The video camera is attached. After a preliminary observation of the abdomen and pelvis, at least two ancillary 5-mm trocars are placed approximately 10 cm lateral to the umbilicus. An additional opening is made, usually in the midline above the symphysis pubis, and a 10-mm trocar is placed to accomodate additional 5- or 10-mm instrument and to remove lymph nodes out of the abdomen. In our experience, the protection provided by the trocar sheath is enough to prevent abdominal wall metastases. Only grossly involved nodes larger that 10-mm wide are removed by an endoscopic bag. The retraction of the bowel may in a few cases require an additional port, either a 4.5 mm for the use of a probe or a closed forceps, or a 10 mm for the optional use of an endoretractor.

The assistant holds the endoscope and the instrument introduced through the left lateral port. The operating table is placed in a 10-degree Trendelenburg position and tilted to the left. The omentum and bowel loops are gently retracted toward the left upper quadrant. This step is essential to maintain the bowel loops out of the field of vision. The aorta is identified under the peritoneum, up to the level of the root of the mesentery. The posterior peritoneum is incised over the lower 5 cm of aorta and the 2 first cm of the right common iliac artery. The left margin of the incision is grasped by the assistant with a forceps. The peritoneum is elevated and retracted laterally to the left side of the patient, in order to create a "wall" between the operative field and the bowel loops. The anterior aspect of the aorta and of the vena cava are identified and freed by blunt dissection. The retroperitoneal space is thus developed beneath the root of the mesentery up to the transverse duodenum. The instrument introduced through the left port, held by the assistant, is then placed in the middle retroperitoneal space, gently lifting the transverse duodenum. The left renal vein is generally identified at this step.

The retroperitoneal space is then developed laterally under the right and left mesocolons, and the psoas muscles are easily reached. The lumbar ureters and ovarian vessels are usually lifted along with the ascending and descending colon, and readily identifiable under the mesocolon. At this point, the assistant is asked to maintain the endoscope in order to visualize the retroperitoneal space only. The anterior aspect of the aorta is freed up to then above the level of the inferior mesenteric artery. The vena cava is identified at the right side of the aorta. Its anterior aspect is easily freed, up to the level then above the level of the right ovarian vein. Its right aspect is identified. In order to dissect free the left renal vein, the dissection is carried out up to the origins of ovarian arteries. Both ovarian arteries may have to be divided once occluded by electro-dessication or clips. This step is essential to allow elevation of the peritoneum and the viscera, providing space for a true panoramic endoscopic view of the retroperitoneal space and giving full access to the left renal vein, from the end of the left ovarian vein to the junction with the vena cava.

The para-aortic cellulolymphatic pads are now ready for removal. The left lateroaortic, the precaval, interaorticocaval, and laterocaval nodal areas may be separately freed from the large vessels and removed.

Throughout the operation, blunt dissection with the closed end of atraumatic forceps or with the tip of the aspiration device (used at the same time to clarify the operative field when necessary) seems to provide the safest way of freeing the cellulolymphatic flaps. Electrosurgery with monopolar scissors or dessication with bipolar electrocautery may also be used. As soon as part of a cellular flap is freed from the great vessels, it may be firmly grasped with a forceps and elevated to show its posterior aspect, overlying the vessels or the prevertebral plane. All of the small vessels going to or coming from the major vessels must be electrodessicated with bipolar forceps or occluded using clips. The lumbar veins are to be identified, particularly beneath the aorta, just in front of the prevertebral fascia. When moderate bleeding occurs, the surgeon must remain calm, and use compression with the tip of a closed atraumatic forceps or the aspiration irrigation cannula. The bleeding stops either spontaneously or after elective haemostasis with clips (vena cava) or electrodessication (aorta).

At the end of the dissection, the supramesenteric interaorticocaval and the upper left aortic lymph nodes are detached from the left renal vein, again using clips to secure haemostasis and lymphostasis. Special care must be given to large veins joining the left renal vein to the lumbar and azygos venous system.

Hemostasis is checked. Sponges are counted. The peritoneum is left open. Fascial incisions 10 mm or larger are closed. Skin incisions are closed using sutures or staples.

EXTRAPERITONEAL PARA–AORTIC LYMPHADENECTOMY

The operation starts as a standard laparoscopy. After the pneumoperitoneum has been created, a 10-mm endoscope is placed at the inferior margin of the umbilicus. An additional 5-mm trocar is placed in the right lower quadrant to accomodate a palpator or a needle for sampling of the peritoneal fluid or a biopsy forceps in case of suspected peritoneal involvement. Additional information concerning the adnexae is obtained.

A 15-mm incision is made 3 to 4 cm medial to the left iliac spine. The skin, fascia, transverse muscles and deep fascia are incised, taking care not to open the peritoneum, which can be avoided if the laparoscopic view is used to check the undersurface of the abdominal wall of the left lower quadrant. The left forefinger of the surgeon is introduced in the incision and frees the peritoneal sac from the deep surface of the muscles of the abdominal wall under laparoscopic monitoring. The dissection is easy in the iliac fossa, and the finger soon reaches the psoas muscle then, more medially, the left common iliac artery. Both landmarks are easily identified with the fingertip as a result of shape (psoas muscle) or beating (common iliac artery). Both landmarks can be safely freed from the peritoneal sac as much as possible: the wider the finger preparation is, the shorter will be the endoscopic dissection. The separation of the peritoneum is more difficult in the cephalic direction, with a thinner and more attached peritoneal sac. It is, however, possible to separate a surface of the abdominal

REFERENCES

1. Querleu D. Laparoscopic paraaortic lymphadenectomy. A preliminary experience. *Gynecol Oncol.* 1993;49:24–29.

2. Querleu D, Leblanc E. Laparoscopic infrarenal node dissection for restaging of carcinomas of the ovary or fallopian tube. *Cancer.* 1994;73:1467–1471.

3. Querleu D, Childers J, Dargent D, eds. *Laparoscopic Surgery in Gynecologic Oncology.* Oxford, UK: Blackwell publishers; 1999.

4. Querleu D, Leblanc E, Cartron G, Narducci F, Ferron G, Martel P. Audit of preoperative and early complications of laparoscopic lymph node dissection in 1000 gynecologic cancer patients. *Amer J Obstet Gynecol.* 2006;195:1287–1292.

5. Occelli B, Narducci F, Lanvin D, Querleu D, Coste E, Castelain B, et al. De novo adhesions with extraperitoneal endosurgical para–aortic lymphadenectomy versus transperitoneal laparoscopic para–aortic lymphadenectomy: A randomized experimental study. *Am J Obstet Gynecol.* 2000;183:529–533.

6. Querleu D, Lanvin D, Elhage A, Leblanc E. An experimental assessment of the learning curve for laparoscopic lymphadenectomy. *Eur J Obstet Gynecol.* 1998;81:55–58.

7. Benedetti-Panici P, Maneschi F, Scambia G, Greggi S, Mancuso S. Anatomic abnormalities of the retroperitoneum for systematic removal of lymph nodes left of the aorta in gynaecologic malignancies. *Obstet Gynecol.* 1994;170:111–116.

8. Kavoussi LR, Sosa E, Chandhoke P, Chodak G, Clayman RV, Hadley R, et al. Complications of laparoscopic pelvic lymph node dissection. *J Urol.* 1993;149:322–325.

9. Köhler C, Klemm P, Schau A, Possover M, Krause N, Tozzi R, et al. Introduction of transperitoneal lymphadenectomy in a gynecologic oncology center: Analysis of 650 laparoscopic pelvic and/or paraaortic transperitoneal lymphadenectomies. *Gynecol Oncol.* 2004;95:52–61.

10. Sonoda Y, Leblanc E, Querleu D, Castelain B, Papageorgiou TH, Lambaudie E, et al. Prospective evaluation of surgical staging of advanced cervical cancer via a laparoscopic extraperitoneal approach. *Gynecol Oncol.* 2003;91:326–331.

11. Benedetti-Panici P, Maneschi F, Scambia G, Greggi S, Cutillo G, D'Andrea G, et al. Lymphatic spread of cervical cancer: An anatomical and pathological study based on 225 radical hysterectomies with systematic pelvic and aortic lymphadenectomy. *Gynecol Oncol.* 1996;62:19–24.

12. Occelli B, Narducci F, Lanvin D, Leblanc E, Querleu D. Learning curves for transperitoneal laparoscopic and extraperitoneal endoscopic paraaortic lymphadenectomy. *J Amer Assoc Gynecol Laparoscopists.* 2000;7:51–53.

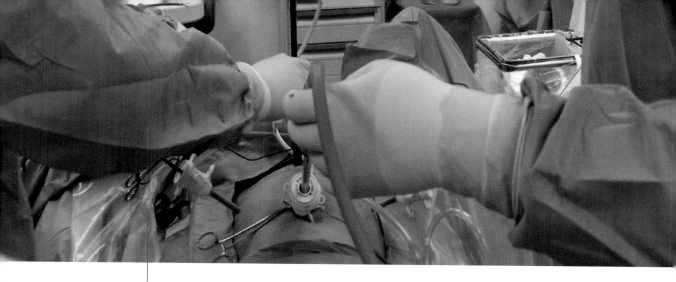

6 LAPAROSCOPY IN THE MORBIDLY OBESE

Katherine A. O'Hanlan

INDICATIONS

Definition and implications of obesity

Obesity is defined as having a body mass index (BMI) (kg/m^2) greater than 30. It leads to multiple organ-specific pathological consequences, particularly for those with intra-abdominal fat accumulation.[1] According to the Women's Health Initiative, women who needed hysterectomy were more likely to have metabolic syndrome (hypertension, diabetes, hypercholesterolemia, obesity) and lower physical activity compared with women who did not have hysterectomy, with subsequently higher risks for cardiovascular events and mortality.[2] Obese women are more likely to develop uterine and ovarian cancers.[3] It is thus important to be able to provide such women with a safe surgical experience when they develop gynecological cancers. Laparoscopic approaches to gynecologic surgery have consistently demonstrated slightly increased operating times, but, more importantly, no increase in complications, less blood loss, less pain, shorter hospital stays, and a quicker return to work for woman regardless of BMI.[4] A total laparoscopic surgical approach for all gynecological procedures, including hysterectomy, adnexectomy, pelvic and aortic lymphadenectomy, omentectomy, and appendectomy is now indicated for most gynecologic patients, including those who are obese, for diagnoses such as recurrent and persistent cervical dysplasia, uterine and endometrial neoplasia,[5] pelvic mass and early ovarian cancer.[6] Total laparoscopic radical hysterectomy is also possible for early cervical cancers and stage II endometrial cancers with clinical spread to the cervix.[7] Laparoscopic approach for exploratory evaluation for exenteration[8] or for performing the exenteration[9] have been reported recently, in small series reports. The applications of laparoscopic surgery in gynecology are constantly expanding with the new technologies and with advancing surgeons' skills.

Physiologic impact of laparoscopy on the obese

The physiology of gynecologic laparoscopy in the obese patient revolves around changes with abdominal insufflation of carbon dioxide (CO_2), or capnoperitoneum, with severe head-down tilt of the operating table, or Trendelenburg position, and with the size of the lower abdominal fat, the pannus, exerting gravitational pressure on the abdominal viscera, vasculature and diaphragm (Figures 6-1 and 6-2). A heavier pannus will require higher intraperitoneal CO_2 pressures and steeper Trendelenburg for optimal pelvic visualization, which can, in turn, result in poor hemodynamic and respiratory functions.[10]

Obesity and pulmonary function during laparoscopy

Compared to preoperative values forced vital capacity (FVC), forced expiratory volume at 1 second (FEV1) and forced expiratory flow at 25% to 75% (FEF 25–75) were found to be reduced by 20% to 30% during and 24 hours after laparoscopic cholecystectomy.[11] Compared to patients having open surgeries, with the attendant incisional pain limiting inspiration, almost one-third laparoscopic patients develop segmental lung collapse, i.e. atelectasis, which is the predominant cause of respiratory acidosis during and after general anesthesia. Of these undergoing surgery, morbidly obese patients develop significantly more atelectasis than do patients with ideal BMI. Moreover in obese patients, atelectasis persists unchanged for more than 24 hours after the surgery, whereas in nonobese patients, lungs re-expand to normal within 24 hours.[12] While atelectasis is thought to be

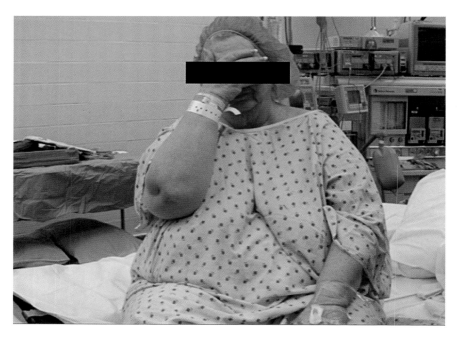

Figure 6-1 ▪ This patient with endometrial carcinoma, grade 1, endometrioid type, weighs 350 pounds, is 5′2″, and has a BMI of 64. A lymph node dissection is not planned for this patient if she is found to have high-risk pathologic features.

caused by the compounding obesity with the immobility from surgery, some cases may also be caused by the slippage of the endotracheal tube, which occurs more often in obese patients as well as more often during laparoscopic cases. In one study, the endotracheal tube slipped in half of laparoscopic patients compared with 20% of laparotomy patients, with most moving downward into the right bronchus, once maximal abdominal insufflation or Trendelenburg was established.[13]

The morbidly obese patient may not tolerate the Trendelenburg position needed for deep pelvic surgery if they have inadequate gas exchange as evidenced by room air oxygen saturations in the low 90% range or a blood gas on room air demonstrating CO_2 retention. Mild to moderately obese patients with severe pulmonary disease may also not tolerate the Trendelenburg position. Those with chronic obstructive pulmonary disease (COPD) whose FEV1/FVC ratio (FEV1 over FVC) is <50% of the normal, or whose FEV1 is <1.2L, or who have pulmonary hypertension or right ventricular failure, or who are on home oxygen risk having

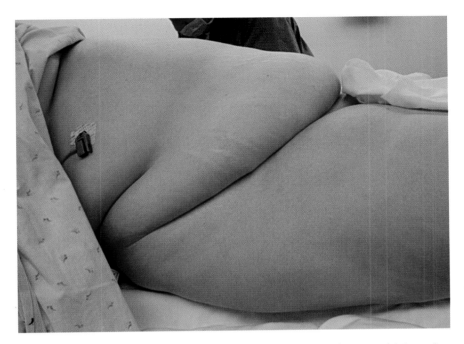

Figure 6-2 ▪ The pannus of this patient folds over the groin and mons pubis in supine position.

inadequate oxygenation and ventilation secondary to ventilation perfusion mismatch.

In preparation for laparoscopic surgery, obese patients should be counseled to optimize their daily exercise and pulmonary function and advised to discontinue any smoking. Obese patients do not routinely need pulmonary function tests, but should undergo testing as a baseline if they already have compromised lung function as with asthma or diagnosed COPD, e.g., from long-term smoking. Low-molecular-weight heparin should be given to reduce the risk of deep vein thrombophlebitis (DVT) and pulmonary embolus (PE).

Capnoperitoneum, even without Trendelenburg, causes significant respiratory changes in the obese. In 15 morbidly obese patients studied prior to gastroplasty, it was found that abdominal insufflation caused a 31% decrease in respiratory compliance, a 17% increase in peak inspiratory pressures, and 32% increase in plateau airway pressures and significant hypercapnia, but no reduction in arterial oxygen saturation.[14] Pulmonary compliance and insufflation pressures returned to baseline values after abdominal deflation. These observed pulmonary alterations in the morbidly obese patients were still well tolerated and confirm that obesity does not compromise ozygenation during laparoscopic surgery.

Postoperative management should thus include immediate ambulationa and vigorous pulmonary toilet to open airways. To facilitate removal of endotracheal phlegm, inspiratory exercise using incentive spirometers, and if needed, supervised respiratory therapist's administration of either solubilized saline or bronchodilators should be employed.

Obesity and cardiovascular function during laparoscopy

Insufflation of the abdomen with CO_2 results in a decrease in cardiac index and stroke volume, and increase in systemic vascular resistance.[15] Venous capacitance decreases progressively during prolonged capnoperitoneum.[16] However, these hemodynamic changes resolve quickly, and are well tolerated. With thorough cardiac preoperative evaluation by stress echocardiography, laparoscopy can be performed safely and is the preferred surgical method in obese patients, even with history of myocardial infarction. Patients with a history of hypertension or cardiovascular disease should receive preoperative β-blockade.

Transumbilical direct trocar placement

Location of the umbilicus over the aorta varies with increasing obesity and poses risk during initial trocar insertion, even with a Veress needle. Use of a blunt, pointed 5-mm trocar inserted directly through a 5-mm incision in the central umbilical apical scar elevated maximally on towel clips has been associated with minimal complications,[17] even in the overweight and obese (O'Hanlan, 2007).[5]

Pneumoperitoneum pressures of 12 to 15 mm Hg is usually the maximum tolerated pressures when the patient is in steep Trendelenburg position.

Hysterectomy and adnexectomy, radical hysterectomy, and lymphadenectomy

Few differences in gynecological surgical parameters are noted for overweight women (BMI 25–30) compared to those with ideal BMI less than 25,[18] but significant differences exist when comparing obese women (BMI > 30) to those with lower BMI. In multiple reports of women with clinical stage I endometrial cancer with BMI up to 60, the operative times were higher for obese patients than those with BMI less than 30 (150 vs. 121 min), but blood loss was lower, postoperative stay were 1 to 3 days, with acceptable or better pelvic node yields of 16 to 21 nodes and similar complications, and disease-free survival.[5,19–22] The usual time for adding a radical pelvic node dissection when patients have high-grade disease or higher than stage IB disease is approximately 50 minutes, with typical nodal yields of 17 to 26 nodes.[23,24] Duration of pelvic lymphadenectomy was independent of BMI,[24] but having a BMI greater than 35 was associated with a decreased laparoscopic lymphadenectomy success rate from 82% to 44%,[25] and in those cases, the laparoscopic procedure took 2 hours longer. Pelvic, common iliac, and paraaortic lymph node counts of 18, 5, and 7 were similar to open nodal yields.[26]

Most obese women with early stage endometrial cancer should be managed with a laparoscopic approach expecting excellent surgical outcomes, shorter hospitalizations and less postoperative pain, and quicker recovery to work than those managed through laparotomy. However, lymphadenectomy may not be possible with BMIs above 50, and external beam extended field pelvic radiation therapy may need to be used more aggressively in these cases.[27] Total laparoscopic radical hysterectomy has been confirmed to offer all the benefits of open surgery for patients with stage IA2 to IB1 cervical cancer, with shorter hospital stay, less blood loss, similar nodal yields, and similar 4-hour durations of surgery when performed by experienced surgeons.[28] Complications in most series occur of approximately 5%,[7] with most training programs implementing fellow participation in the surgery.[29] A 1-day hospital stay for both simple and radical hysterectomy, with and without node dissections, is now standard.[23,30]

Paraaortic lymphadenectomy

Laparoscopic urologists confirm that morbid obesity can limit access to the retroperitoneum, but the extraperitoneal rather than transperitoneal approach is still optimal for surgery on the kidney and nodes for obese patients.[31] Using an extraperitoneal laparoscopic approach for inframesenteric aortic node dissection on 76 women, an average of 14 aortic nodes were obtained; however, three patients were converted to open laparotomy because of the limitations from obesity and three because of the peritoneal tears.[32] Right-sided para-aortic, left-sided inframesenteric, and left-sided infrarenal lymphadenectomy added a mean of 28 to 62 minutes, with nodal yields independent of the patient's BMI.[24] Most intraoperative and postoperative complication rates involve vessel, urologic, or bowel injury and occur in less than 5% of patients, regardless of BMI.[5] Most surgeons demonstrate a learning curve in performing laparoscopic lymphadenectomy and include patients with higher BMI as their experience accrues.[24]

Appendectomy, omentectomy, and staging

Appendectomy and omentectomy are indicated in the staging of early ovarian carcinoma because occult metastasis to these organs occurs in approximately one third of patients with clinically early ovarian cancer. Laparoscopy is the preferred approach for acute appendicitis, especially for the obese.[33] Laparoscopic appendectomy for staging of early ovarian cancer, or for prophylaxis against appendicitis confers no added time to the primary procedure, and does not add to the hospital stay or complication rate[34] (Figure 6-3). The age-adjusted incidence of acute appendicitis after age 40 is similar to that of ovarian cancer, lending reason to perform incidental appendectomy during all pelvic laparoscopy cases, when feasible.[34]

Omentectomy in the obese is carried out carefully following the margin of the colon, using a sealing cutting device such as the Ligasure, Enseal,

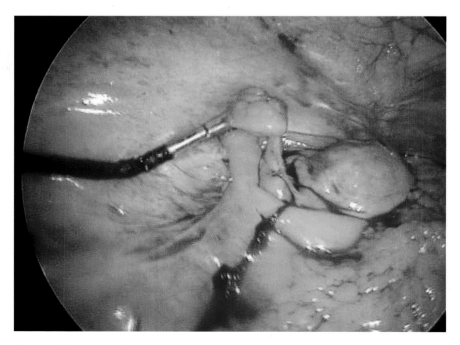

Figure 6-3 ■ Appendectomy in the obese patient is safe and feasible in cases of early ovarian cancer, or as prophylaxis against appendicitis.

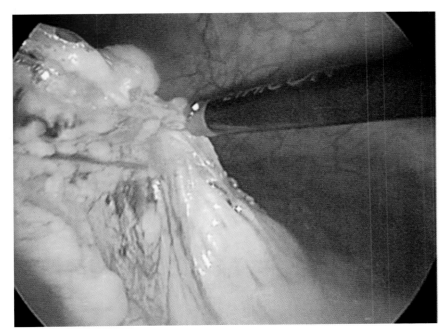

Figure 6-4 ■ Omentectomy can be performed by following the margin of the bowel.

or Harmonic Scalpel.[6] By identifying the descending colon margin of origin of the omentum, and incising 1 to 2 cm away from the colon margin, following the edge up to the splenic flexure, across the transverse colon, to end at the margin of the omentum on the ascending colon, surgeons can avoid losing their bearings in the very large 2-kg omenta such as some obese women posess[6] (Figure 6-4).

Exenteration

Exenteration for recurrent cervical and endometrial carcinoma has been reported in small series and is the current frontier of laparoscopic gynecologic cancer surgery.[35–37]

Contraindications and prevention of complications in the obese patient

Limits of BMI. Predictions of need to convert to laparotomy because of the patients' size, based on predictions from computed tomographic

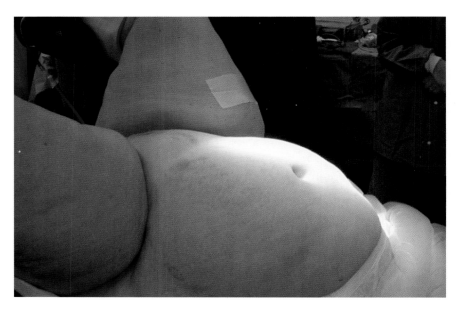

Figure 6-5 ▪ Demonstration of mobility of pannus upward in steep Trendelenburg position.

estimates of intra-abdominal visceral fat were accurate in a study of 151 women with endometrial cancer.[38] This study demonstrates that patients with hip adiposity were more easily completed than those with abdominal adiposity. Assessment of the obese patient in supine Trendelenburg position on the office examining table can give an idea of how well the distribution of adiposity will lend itself to laparoscopic surgery (Figure 6-5).

Pulmonary disease

Laparoscopic surgery is quite safe in morbidly obese patients with normal respiratory mechanics[14] and has been performed safely in 14 patients on the lung transplant waiting list with end-stage lung disease.[39] In a study of morbidly obese patients with COPD, the airway resistance and peak inspiratory pressures were increased throughout the insufflation and could be improved with a 20-degree reverse Trendelenburg position.[40] Cardiac function studies showed no clinically significant changes in this study of patients in supine position; however, gynecological patients are in steep Trendelenburg position, which causes respiratory acidosis, and worsens ventilatory compliance, increasing inspiratory pressures, raising

CO_2 levels in the blood. During the progress of surgery on obese patients in steep Trendelenburg, whenever the CO_2 levels become elevated, the first compensatory step is increasing the minute volume of ventilation,[15] and then, if needed, by intermittent reduction of the depth of the tilt, by lowering the pressure of the capnoperitoneum, or by initiating periods of complete deflation of the capnoperitoneum with supine position until the CO_2 pressures are "breathed down" to the high normal range. Then reinstitution of capnoperitoneum and Trendelenburg allows continuation of the surgery, until hypercapnea demands another period of resolution. This cycle can be safely repeated until the surgery is completed.

Cardiac disease

In a detailed study of morbidly obese patients undergoing cholecystectomy, monitoring with noninvasive hemodynamic measurements including cardiac index, mean arterial pressure, and heart rate, calculated systemic vascular resistance and mean arterial pressure recorded every 5 min and at specific predetermined times, it was revealed that generally, obese patients were hemodynamically as stable as their nonobese counterparts.[41] Patients with ischemic left ventricular dysfunction and with significant aortic stenosis were observed by transesophageal echocardiography to withstand laparoscopic cholecystectomy without cardiac complications.[42] One patient with congestive heart failure and an ejection fraction of 15% was observed to tolerate laparoscopic cholecystectomy.[43] Cardiac patients should be medically optimized and intra-abdominal pressures and surgical times minimized, anticipating minimal risk to the patient undergoing laparoscopic procedures.

Obesity and deep vein DVT and PE

Obesity, age over 40 years, capnoperitoneum, Trendelenburg position, and long operations are all risk factors for DVT.[44,45] In a meta-analysis of over 7639 cancer patients having surgery, the incidence of DVT/PE was found to be reduced from 35% to 7% by use of low-molecular-weight heparin.[45] Current surgical care standards require both preoperative and postoperative prophylaxis with high-dose low-molecular-weight heparin, 40 mg every 12 hours[46] and early ambulation, continued throughout the hospitalization until full mobility is regained, longer for patients with prior DVT.[45] In one large series of obese patients undergoing laparoscopic digestive surgeries, using preoperative doses of low-molecular-weight heparin, the incidence of DVT was 0.33% and there were no cases of PE.[47]

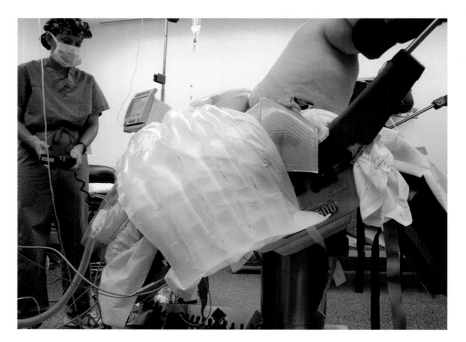

Figure 6-6 ■ Demonstration of tilt of table to approximately 45 degrees Trendelenburg.

Setup, patient positioning, and equipment

Any time that pelvic access may be necessary during laparoscopic surgery, a modified lithotomy position is used. Trendelenberg position to 45 degrees must be possible for adequate visualization for pelvic procedures, especially in women with higher BMI (Figure 6-6). Ascertain that the operating room table will tilt adequately ahead of time. Arms must be tucked in by the patient's side with protection of the fingers by wrapping them to the lateral thigh. Plexiglas "sleds" are placed under the mid-arm beneath the cushion of the table extending the effective width of the table, since obese patients are usually wider than the tables themselves. The elbows are cushioned with gel pads to prevent ulnar nerve injury (Figure 6-7). To prevent slippage of the patient up the table in Trendelenburg, shoulder bolsters are clipped to the sidebar of the table with gel pads on the shoulder to prevent nerve injury (Figure 6-8). Legs are nearly extended at the hips, and flexed 80 degrees at the knees. To facilitate thermoregulation, a warmed air device is placed over the patient's upper torso and head and the legs are wrapped in a blanket.

Direct umbilical trocar entry into an uninsufflated abdomen is easiest.[4] Regular or extra-long trocars are inserted and sutured in place to prevent

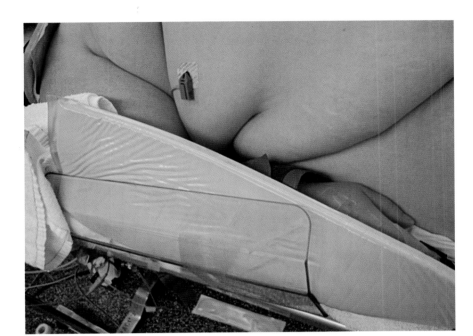

Figure 6-7 ■ The Plexiglas sleds extend the support of the table, and protect the arms. Gel pads are placed under the elbows to cushion the ulnar nerve. Hands are wrapped in a towel and taped to the thigh to prevent injury to the fingers.

slippage of the tip out of the peritoneal cavity. Rather than aiming trocars perpendicularly into the abdominal cavity, we aim the trocars into the pelvis to avoid stretch of the fascia and reduce hernia risk.[48] Retraction of the viscera to enable pelvic surgery is sometimes needed. In these cases, a 10-mm umbilical trocar is inserted through which a 10-mm expandable endoscopic retractor can be used. An additional 5-mm port is placed approximately 6 to 8 mm below the umbilical port in the midline for the lighted videoscope.

Pre- and postopertive management

Obese women requiring hysterectomy are more likely to have metabolic syndrome[2] and need special consideration regarding preoperative evaluation and testing, as well as postoperative systemic health management issues. Obese women are also less likely to be in compliance with standard screening tests[49] and require careful preoperative evaluation of cardiac and pulmonary function.

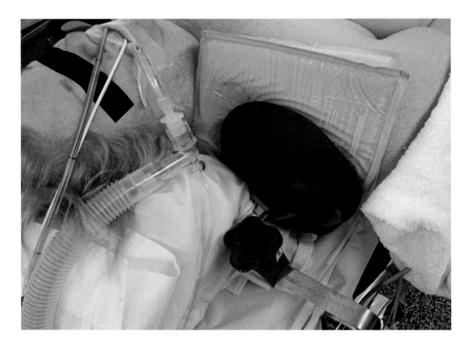

Figure 6-8 ■ This shoulder bolster is centered on the acromion process, over a gel pad, and clipped to the sidebar of the table to prevent upward slippage during steep Trendelenburg.

Obese women may be on multiple medications for metabolic syndrome, most of which can be continued throughout their brief stay in the hospital for laparoscopic surgery. Anticholesterolemics can be continued or discontinued briefly without ill effect. Antihypertensives including the ace inhibitors and β-blockers should be continued perioperatively with a sip of water. Oral hypoglycemic agents and insulin should be administered on the day of surgery at half dose, withholding all glucose in the intravenous solutions. An insulin drip may be necessary during the surgery. High-volume gastric acidity observed in obese patients should be prevented with H_2 blockers, such as famotidine or pantoprazole.

CONTRAINDICATIONS

The limitations of a laparoscopic approach emanate from patient factors, equipment factors, and the surgeon's experience. All prior abdominal surgeries should be reviewed for the possibility of severe adhesions, which can preclude a safe laparoscopic approach. A prior midline incision is not a contraindication for laparoscopic treatment, but does suggest consideration for employing a left subcostal insertion of the first trocar.

CONCLUSION

Total laparoscopic simple and radical hysterectomy/adnexectomy with indicated pelvic and aortic lymphadenectomy, appendectomy and omentectomy are all feasible and safe for patients with high BMI. This approach confers significant benefits in reduced blood loss, length of hospital stay, and confers a similar efficacy and complication rate, even when stratified by BMI. Limitations to node dissections may be seen with BMI greater than 50. The clinical considerations reviewed above and undertaken for the obese patient with a gynecological malignancy can reduce complications and optimize outcomes, regardless of BMI.

REFERENCES

1. Lean ME. Pathophysiology of obesity. *Proc Nutr Soc.* 2000;59(3):331–336.
2. Howard BV, Kuller L, Langer R, et al. Risk of cardiovascular disease by hysterectomy status, with and without oophorectomy: The Women's Health Initiative Observational Study. *Circulation.* 2005;111(12):1462–1470.
3. Anderson B, Connor JP, Andrews JI, et al. Obesity and prognosis in endometrial cancer. *Am J Obstet Gynecol.* 1996;174(4):1171–1178.
4. O'Hanlan KA, Lopez L, Dibble SL, Garnier AC, Huang GS, Leuchtenberger M. Total laparoscopic hysterectomy: Body mass index and outcomes. *Obstet Gynecol.* 2003;102(6):1384–1392.
5. O'Hanlan KA, Dibble SL, Fisher DT. Total laparoscopic hysterectomy for uterine pathology: Impact of body mass index on outcomes. *Gynecol Oncol.* 2006;103(3):938–941.
6. O'Hanlan KA, Huang GS, Lopez L, Garnier AC. Selective incorporation of total laparoscopic hysterectomy for adnexal pathology and body mass index. *Gynecol Oncol.* 2004;93(1):137–143.
7. Ramirez PT, Slomovitz BM, Soliman PT, Coleman RL, Levenback C. Total laparoscopic radical hysterectomy and lymphadenectomy: the M.D. Anderson Cancer Center experience. *Gynecol Oncol.* 2006;102(2):252–255.

8. Plante M, Roy M. Operative laparoscopy prior to a pelvic exenteration in patients with recurrent cervical cancer. *Gynecol Oncol.* 1998;69(2):94-99.

9. Lin MY, Fan EW, Chiu AW, Tian YF, Wu MP, Liao AC. Laparoscopy-assisted transvaginal total exenteration for locally advanced cervical cancer with bladder invasion after radiotherapy. *J Endourol.* 2004;18(9):867-870.

10. Stany MP, Winter WE, 3rd, Dainty L, Lockrow E, Carlson JW. Laparoscopic exposure in obese high-risk patients with mechanical displacement of the abdominal wall. *Obstet Gynecol.* 2004;103(2):383-386.

11. Ravimohan SM, Kaman L, Jindal R, Singh R, Jindal SK. Postoperative pulmonary function in laparoscopic versus open cholecystectomy: Prospective, comparative study. *Indian J Gastroenterol.* 2005;24(1):6-8.

12. Eichenberger A, Proietti S, Wicky S, et al. Morbid obesity and postoperative pulmonary atelectasis: An underestimated problem. *Anesth Analg.* 2002;95(6):1788-1792.

13. Ezri T, Hazin V, Warters D, Szmuk P, Weinbroum AA. The endotracheal tube moves more often in obese patients undergoing laparoscopy compared with open abdominal surgery. *Anesth Analg.* 2003;96(1):278-282.

14. Dumont L, Mattys M, Mardirosoff C, Vervloesem N, Alle JL, Massaut J. Changes in pulmonary mechanics during laparoscopic gastroplasty in morbidly obese patients. *Acta Anaesthesiol Scand.* 1997;41(3):408-413.

15. Stone J, Dyke L, Fritz P, et al. Hemodynamic and hormonal changes during pneumoperitoneum and trendelenburg positioning for operative gynecologic laparoscopy surgery. *Prim Care Update Ob Gyns.* 1998;5(4):155.

16. Maillo CL, Martin E, Lopez J, et al. Effect of pneumoperitoneum on venous hemodynamics during laparoscopic cholecystectomy. Influence of patients' age and time of surgery. *Med Clin (Barc).* Mar 15 2003;120(9):330-334.

17. Jacobson MT, Helmy M, Smith KS, Nezhat CH, Nezhat F, Nezhat CR. Transumbilical direct trocar entry for operative videolaparoscopy. *Obstet Gynecol.* 2000;95(4 Suppl 1):S33.

18. Bai SW, Lim JH, Kim JY, Chung KA, Kim SK, Park KH. Relationship between obesity and the risk of gynecologic laparoscopy in Korean women. *J Am Assoc Gynecol Laparosc.* 2002;9(2):165-169.

19. Caquant F, Mas-Calvet M, Turbelin C, et al. Endometrial cancer by laparoscopy and vaginal approach in the obese patient. *Bull Cancer.* Apr 1 2006;93(4):402-406.

20. Eltabbakh GH, Shamonki MI, Moody JM, Garafano LL. Hysterectomy for obese women with endometrial cancer: Laparoscopy or laparotomy? *Gynecol Oncol.* 2000;78(3 Pt 1):329-335.

21. Ghezzi F, Cromi A, Bergamini V, et al. Laparoscopic management of endometrial cancer in nonobese and obese women: A consecutive series. *J Minim Invasive Gynecol.* 2006;13(4):269-275.

22. Heinberg EM, Crawford BL III, Weitzen SH, Bonilla DJ. Total laparoscopic hysterectomy in obese versus nonobese patients. *Obstet Gynecol.* 2004;103(4):674-680.

23. O'Hanlan KA, Pinto RA, O'Holleran MS. Total laparoscopic hysterectomy with and without lymph node dissection for uterine neoplasia. *J Minim Invasive Gynecol.* 2007;14(4):449-452.

24. Kohler C, Klemm P, Schau A, et al. Introduction of transperitoneal lymphadenectomy in a gynecologic oncology center: Analysis of 650 laparoscopic pelvic and/or paraaortic transperitoneal lymphadenectomies. *Gynecol Oncol.* 2004;95(1): 52-61.

25. Scribner DR Jr, Walker JL, Johnson GA, McMeekin DS, Gold MA, Mannel RS. Laparoscopic pelvic and paraaortic lymph node dissection in the obese. *Gynecol Oncol.* 2002;84(3):426-430.

26. Scribner DR Jr, Walker JL, Johnson GA, McMeekin SD, Gold MA, Mannel RS. Laparoscopic pelvic and paraaortic lymph node dissection: Analysis of the first 100 cases. *Gynecol Oncol.* 2001;82(3):498-503.

27. Greven KM, Corn BW. Endometrial cancer. *Curr Probl Cancer.* 1997;21(2):65-127.

28. Nezhat F, Mahdavi A, Nagarsheth NP. Total laparoscopic radical hysterectomy and pelvic lymphadenectomy using harmonic shears. *J Minim Invasive Gynecol.* 2006;13(1):20-25.

29. Zakashansky K, Chuang L, Gretz H, Nagarsheth NP, Rahaman J, Nezhat FR. A case-controlled study of total laparoscopic radical hysterectomy with pelvic lymphadenectomy versus radical abdominal hysterectomy in a fellowship training program. *Int J Gynecol Cancer.* 2007.

30. Ramirez PT, Slomovitz BM, Soliman PT, Coleman RL, Levenback C. Total laparoscopic radical hysterectomy and lymphadenectomy: The M. D. Anderson Cancer Center experience. *Gynecol Oncol.* 2006;102(2):252-255.

31. Gong EM, Orvieto MA, Lyon MB, Lucioni A, Gerber GS, Shalhav AL. Analysis of impact of body mass index on outcomes of laparoscopic renal surgery. *Urology.* 2007;69(1):38-43.

32. Nagao S, Fujiwara K, Kagawa R, et al. Feasibility of extraperitoneal laparoscopic para-aortic and common iliac lymphadenectomy. *Gynecol Oncol.* 2006;103(2): 732-735.

33. Enochsson L, Hellberg A, Rudberg C, et al. Laparoscopic vs. open appendectomy in overweight patients. *Surg Endosc.* 2001;15(4):387-392.

34. O'Hanlan KA, Fisher DT, O'Holleran MS. 257 incidental appendectomies during total laparoscopic hysterectomy. *JSLS.* 2007;11(4):428-431.

35. Uzan C, Rouzier R, Castaigne D, Pomel C. Laparoscopic pelvic exenteration for cervical cancer relapse: Preliminary study. *J Gynecol Obstet Biol Reprod (Paris).* 2006;35(2):136-145.

36. Pomel C, Rouzier R, Pocard M, et al. Laparoscopic total pelvic exenteration for cervical cancer relapse. *Gynecol Oncol.* 2003;91(3):616-618.

37. Puntambekar S, Kudchadkar RJ, Gurjar AM, et al. Laparoscopic pelvic exenteration for advanced pelvic cancers: A review of 16 cases. *Gynecol Oncol.* 2006;102(3):513-516.

38. Palomba S, Zupi E, Russo T, et al. Presurgical assessment of intraabdominal visceral fat in obese patients with early-stage endometrial cancer treated with laparoscopic approach: Relationships with early laparotomic conversions. *J Minim Invasive Gynecol.* 2007;14(2):195–201.

39. Linden PA, Gilbert RJ, Yeap BY, et al. Laparoscopic fundoplication in patients with end-stage lung disease awaiting transplantation. *J Thorac Cardiovasc Surg.* 2006;131(2):438–446.

40. Salihoglu Z, Demiroluk S, Dikmen Y. Respiratory mechanics in morbid obese patients with chronic obstructive pulmonary disease and hypertension during pneumoperitoneum. *Eur J Anaesthesiol.* 2003;20(8):658–661.

41. Aloni Y, Evron S, Ezri T, et al. Morbidly obese patients are hemodynamically stable during laparoscopic surgery: A thoracic bioimpedance study. *J Clin Monit Comput.* 2006;20(4):261–266.

42. Danzig V, Krska Z, Demes R, Danzigova Z, Linhart A, Kittnar O. Hemodynamic response to laparoscopic cholecystectomy—impacts of increased afterload and ischemic dysfunction of the left ventricle. *Physiol Res.* 2005;54(4):377–385.

43. Jones PE, Sayson SC, Koehler DC. Laparoscopic cholecystectomy in a cardiac transplant candidate with an ejection fraction of less than 15%. *JSLS.* 1998;2(1):89–92.

44. Holzheimer RG. Laparoscopic procedures as a risk factor of deep venous thrombosis, superficial ascending thrombophlebitis and pulmonary embolism—case report and review of the literature. *Eur J Med Res.* 29 2004;9(9):417–422.

45. Leonardi MJ, McGory ML, Ko CY. A systematic review of deep venous thrombosis prophylaxis in cancer patients: Implications for improving quality. *Ann Surg Oncol.* 2007;14(2):929–936.

46. Clagett GP, Anderson FA, Jr., Heit J, Levine MN, Wheeler HB. Prevention of venous thromboembolism. *Chest.* 1995;108(4 Suppl):312S–334S.

47. Catheline JM, Turner R, Gaillard JL, Rizk N, Champault G. Thromboembolism in laparoscopic surgery: Risk factors and preventive measures. *Surg Laparosc Endosc Percutan Tech.* 1999;9(2):135–139.

48. Nezhat C, Nezhat F, Seidman DS. Incisional hernias after operative laparoscopy. *J Laparoendosc Adv Surg Tech A.* 1997;7(2):111–115.

49. Wee CC, McCarthy EP, Davis RB, Phillips RS. Screening for cervical and breast cancer: Is obesity an unrecognized barrier to preventive care? *Ann Intern Med.* 2000;132(9):697–704.

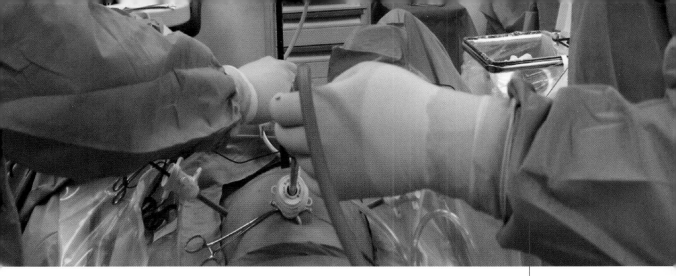

LAPAROSCOPIC BOWEL RESECTION, ANASTOMOSIS, AND ILEOSTOMY/COLOSTOMY

7

Nimesh P. Nagarsheth, David S. Bub, and Farr Nezhat

INDICATIONS

In general indications for laparoscopic bowel resection and anastomosis and/or ostomy formation in the gynecologic oncology patient are the same as indications for traditional open surgery. The most common indications are as follows:

- Primary cytoreduction of ovarian, primary peritoneal, or fallopian tube cancer.[1-4]
- Management of malignant obstruction by small or large bowel bypass or creation of diverting stoma.[2,3]

- Secondary cytoreduction of recurrent ovarian, primary peritoneal, or fallopian tube cancer.[5,6]
- Pelvic exenteration for selected primary or recurrent cervical, endometrial, vaginal, and vulvar cancers.[7-10]
- Secondary cytoreduction (nonexenterative procedures) of recurrent endometrial cancer or uterine sarcomas.[11-13]
- Rectosigmoid colon resection for the management of severe pelvic endometriosis.[14-17]

CONTRAINDICATIONS

Although both absolute and relative contraindications exist to performing laparoscopic bowel surgery, we believe that the ultimate decision as to whether or not to proceed with a laparoscopic approach must be made on a case-by-case basis by the responsible surgeon. The list provided below includes the most common absolute and relative contraindications.

- Medical conditions preventing pneumoperitoneum such as severe cardiovascular compromise.
- Previous abdominal surgery with extensive adhesive disease.
- Diffuse large volume intra-abdominal metastatic disease.
- Morbid obesity.

SETUP, PATIENT POSITIONING, AND EQUIPMENT

We typically perform laparoscopic bowel resections in conjunction with other procedures related to cancer staging and/or cytoreduction. Therefore, we prefer a standard approach regarding setup and positioning for our patients undergoing laparoscopic procedures. First, patients are positioned in the dorsal lithotomy position with adjustable stirrups. Deep vein thrombosis prophylaxis with sequential pneumatic compression devices is performed in all those patients who do not have a contraindication to application of these devices.[18] In selected "higher-risk" patients, a more intense prophylaxis regimen which includes the addition of low-molecular-weight heparin or unfractionated heparin is performed.[19]

The operating room setup is arranged to the surgeon's preference and varies according to the procedures being performed. Nonetheless, for patients undergoing pelvic surgery, we prefer a standard setup of one or two video monitors placed at the foot of the bed. Monitors may be rotated to the patient's right or left side as different quadrants of the abdomen are explored (Figure 7-1). Standard instrument tables and a separate Mayo stand

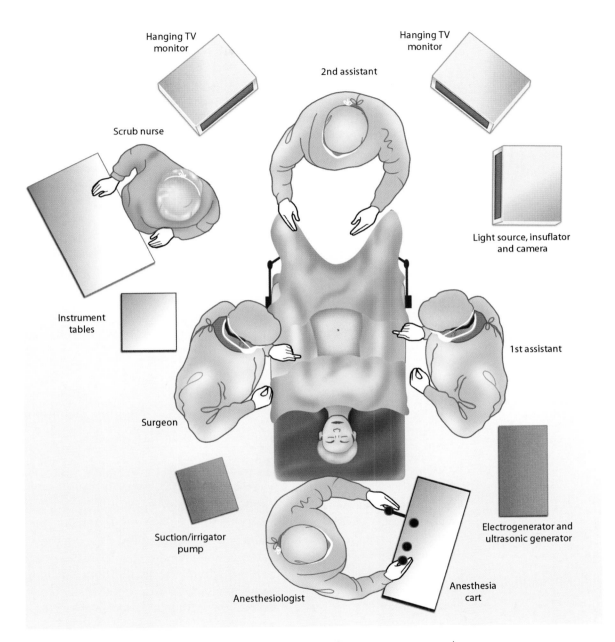

Figure 7-1 ■ Operating room setup demonstrating location of instruments, personnel, and equipment when working on pelvic-directed surgical resections. For upper abdominal resections, rotation of monitors, equipment, and personnel to the patient's right or left side may be appropriate.

for a dilation and curettage tray as well as a separate Mayo stand with laparoscopic bowel graspers, appropriate stapling devices, and equipment for laparoscopic suturing (intracorporeal and/or extracorporeal) are available as necessary.

In addition to standard laparoscopic equipment (hydrodissection pump with suction irrigator probe, bipolar and unipolar cautery, etc.), stapling devices are also made available. Although several different brands of staplers now exist, the three general categories of staplers that we have found useful in laparoscopic bowel surgery include the thoracoabdominal linear stapling instruments (extracorporeal stapling), gastrointestinal anastomosis stapling instruments (both intracorporeal and extracorporeal stapling), and the end-to-end anastomosis (EEA) stapling instruments (preferred for rectosigmoid colon anastomosis). A separate rectal tray including a sigmoidoscope, EEA stapling devices, and bulb syringe with diluted betadine is provided when rectosigmoid colon anastomosis is anticipated. We prefer the use of endoscopic stapling devices when performing intracorporeal bowel division and anastomosis; however, traditional suture techniques of bowel closure and anastomosis in one or two layers using polyglactin 910 (Vicryl) suture (or other appropriate preferred suture materials) are also appropriate for the skilled laparoscopic surgeon.[20]

PREOPERATIVE AND POSTOPERATIVE MANAGEMENT

Patients undergoing planned or anticipated bowel procedures are counseled and consented preoperatively about the possibility of requiring a temporary or permanent ostomy. An ostomy nurse or other qualified individual should carefully examine the patient in a variety of positions (lying, sitting, and standing) and determine and mark the optimal location for a potential ostomy on both sides. In general, the site should be overlying the rectus muscle, accessible to the patient (both visually and manually), and not fall within the waistline or skin crease (which would make securing of an appliance difficult). In an ideal setting, a patient may wear an appliance preoperatively for a few days as a "dry run" to determine the adequacy of the proposed site.

The notion that a preoperative mechanical bowel preparation is necessary to decrease the incidence of postoperative wound complications and anastomotic leak has been surgical dogma for the decades. The first suggestion that a mechanical bowel preparation is not mandatory in patient's undergoing bowel surgery originated from the trauma literature, which demonstrated primary colonic anastomosis could be performed safely in trauma patients who did not undergo preoperative cleansing.[21,22]

Recently, several reports have compared elective colon resection with and without mechanical bowel preparation. Bucher et al.[23] (2004) performed a meta-analysis of seven prospective trials for elective colorectal surgery without bowel preparation including more than 1100 patients. There was a higher incidence of anastomotic leak in the patients undergoing mechanical bowel preparation (5.6%) versus no mechanical bowel preparation (2.8%). Hypotheses for the increased rate of bowel leak include patient dehydration, inflammatory changes to the bowel mucosa, and spillage of liquid stool. There is even suggestion that the use of a bowel preperation can lead to increased rates of intraabdominal sepsis postoperatively.[24] Finally, mechanical bowel preparation has not been shown to improve appropriateness of the surgical field or handling of bowel with laparoscopic instruments in patients undergoing gynecologic laparoscopy.[25]

The routine use of nasogastric decompression in the postoperative period is not recommended. The use of nasogastric tube leads to a longer time to flatus, longer hospital stay, and increased risk of pulmonary complication without improvement in patient comfort or decreased risk of anastomotic leak.[26] Standardized perioperative protocols can lead to quicker resumption of oral feeding and shorter length of stay.[27,28]

Technique

Advances in laparoscopic surgical instrumentation has greatly facilitated laparoscopic bowel surgery. Division of the bowel mesentery can be safely and rapidly performed using an endoscopic intestinal stapler, ultrasonic shears, or bipolar vessel sealing system. Devices differ mainly on their size and the diameter of the vessel they are able to ligate. The ultrasonic shears require a 5-mm trocar and the newer versions of this instrument have been approved for sealing vessels 5 mm in diameter. Endostaplers require careful dissection of the vessels, and require a 12-mm trocar. Bipolar vessel sealing systems come as a 5- or 10-mm instrument and can ligate and divide vessels up to 7 mm in diameter with minimal lateral thermal spread. The choice of instrument to divide the bowel mesentery is clearly up to surgeon preference; however, for adequate lymph node retrieval in colorectal cancer, the American Society of Colon and Rectal Surgery mandates intracorporeal vessel ligation.

Additional techniques and devices are utilized for specific operating conditions. The use of a hand-assist device, either the Lap Disc (Ethicon Endosurgery) or GelPort (Applied Medical) can significantly facilitate bowel resection especially when working with inflamed intestine. By having a hand inside the abdomen, the operating surgeon has increased tactile sensation, and can perform blunt mobilization of the colon manually. Hand-assisted laparoscopy (HALS) has shorter operating times and is a valuable tool when working with inexperienced assistants. Regardless of the instruments used, we encourage the interested surgeon to begin with a standardized technique. When performing bowel resection for colorectal cancer, the following principles are mandated by the colorectal and laparoscopic surgical societies. Similar principles can be extrapolated to the management of gynecologic cancers.

1. Intracorporeal ligation of the mesentery.
2. Wound protection when removing the specimen.
3. Extracorporeal small bowel or colonic anastomosis when feasible.

As one gains experience with the above principles, more advanced techniques such as intracorporeal anastomosis can be performed.

After abdominal insufflation, additional working ports are placed (Figure 7-2). Ports should be placed about a hands breadth apart to allow for adequate range of motion without interacting with an adjacent instrument. In most instances, we use two lower abdominal ports placed 2 fingerbreadths medial and superior from the anterior superior iliac spine. Additional ports are placed in the upper abdomen either in the left or right upper quadrant to help triangulate in our operating field. For example, if performing a right hemicolectomy, we will use a 10- to 12-mm port in the left lower quadrant for a ligasure device or endostapler, and conversely in the right lower quadrant if working on the left colon. Alternatively, we have found a 10- to 12-mm midline suprapubic port (instead of in the lateral position) can perform a similar function while allowing access to the deeper pelvis.

Small bowel bypass

In most cases, an intracorporeal anastomosis is not needed because the portion of bowel to be removed is externalized before resection. However, an intracorporeal anastomosis may be useful in a bowel bypass caused by malignant obstruction. It would be rare to use laparoscopic technique in a

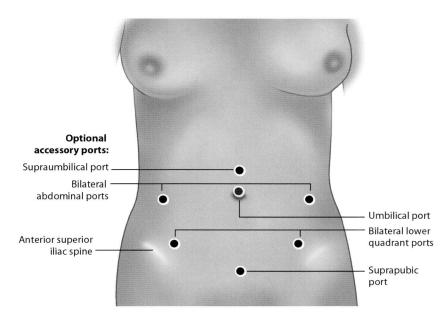

Optional accessory ports:
Supraumbilical port
Bilateral abdominal ports
Anterior superior iliac spine
Umbilical port
Bilateral lower quadrant ports
Suprapubic port

Figure 7-2 ▪ Port placement for gynecologic oncology procedures including laparoscopic bowel resections typically includes an umbilical port (5 or 10 mm), two lower quadrant ports (5 mm each), and a suprapubic port (12 mm). Additional ports (including lateral abdominal or supraumbilical ports) can be added or substituted as needed.

patient with a frozen abdomen caused by carcinomatosis; however, these techniques are standardized and may be helpful in unusual circumstances.

After careful inspection of the bowel (Figure 7-3), the two loops of bowel are isolated inside the abdomen. If division of a bowel segment is required, it can be performed using the endoscopic gastrointestinal stapling device (Figure 7-4) and division of the bowel mesentery can be performed using the ultrasonic shears (Figure 7-5). A stay suture (the "crotch stitch") of 3-0 Vicryl is placed allowing for stabilization of these loops (Figure 7-6). A small antimesenteric enterotomy is made in each bowel loop using the electrocautery or ultrasonic cautery device (Figure 7-7). With the bowel loops held in place, an intracorporeal anastomosis is accomplished by performing 1 or 2 fires of the endoscopic gastrointestinal stapler creating a side-to-side anastomosis. Care must be taken to keep the mesentery rotated inferiorly and not included in the jaws of the stapler (Figure 7-8). The combined enterotomies are then closed using a running two-layer technique by laparoscopic suturing technique, or closed by using the endoscopic stapling device (Figure 7-9).

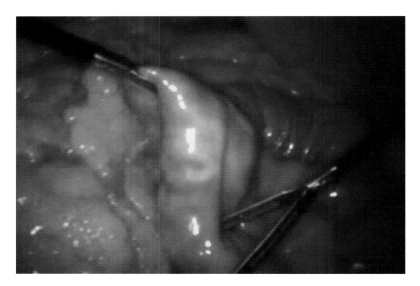

Figure 7-3 ■ The small and large bowel (and bowel mesentery) is routinely inspected during each case. For small bowel inspection, two atraumatic graspers are used to run the small bowel from the ligament of Treitz to the terminal ileum. This procedure can be performed by one individual or can be performed by two individuals working together in a synchronized fashion.

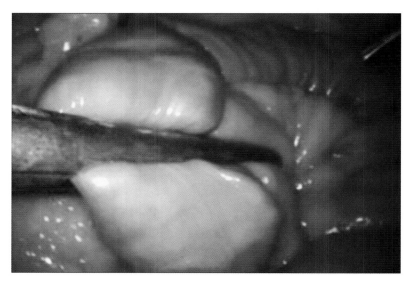

Figure 7-4 ■ Although small bowel resection is not routinely performed during small bowel bypass, the technique of intracorporeal division is demonstrated here using the endoscopic gastrointestinal stapling device.

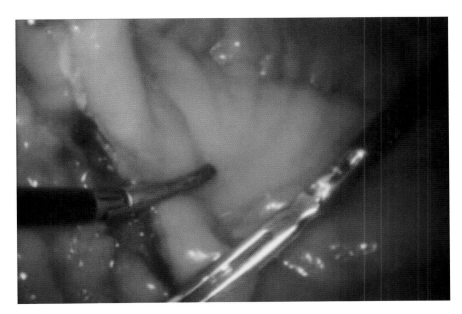

Figure 7-5 ▪ The small bowel mesentery is divided using the harmonic shears.

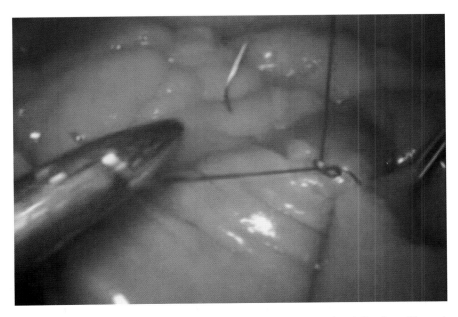

Figure 7-6 ▪ A "crotch stitch" is placed in order to align proximal and distal small bowel segments in preparation for a side-to-side anastomosis.

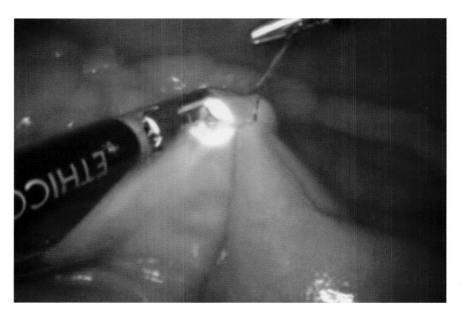

Figure 7-7 ▪ Enterotomies are created in the small bowel using the harmonic shears.

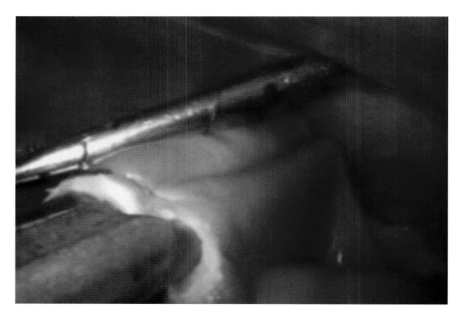

Figure 7-8 ▪ Intracorporeal side-to-side anastomosis of small bowel is performed using the endoscopic gastrointestinal stapling device. Two fires of the stapling device are performed (one in a proximal direction and one in a distal direction) to ensure an adequate lumen.

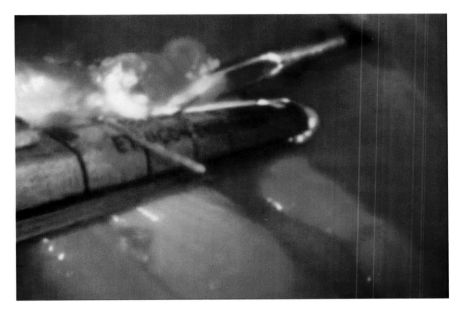

Figure 7-9 ▪ Closure of enterotomy and completion of small bowel bypass anastomosis is accomplished by the use of the gastrointestinal stapling device.

Loop ileostomy

Laparoscopic loop ileostomy is performed in a fashion similar to an open technique. First, if necessary, the small bowel is mobilized by division of peritoneal attachments in the region of the ileocolic junction by using a combination of both blunt and sharp dissection and using the bipolar vessel sealing device (Figure 7-10). Then, a disc of skin is removed using the electrosurgical unit at a previously marked site (see the preoperative management section for determining ostomy locations). The dissection is carried down bluntly to the fascia and a cruciate incision is made approximately 2 fingerbreadths in diameter. The rectus muscles are bluntly separated and posterior sheath and peritoneum are entered sharply (Figure 7-11). After creating the abdominal defect, the loop of ileum is brought up through the stoma site and a window is made in the bowel mesentery just underneath the bowel wall (between vasa recta) and a glass or plastic rod is placed through the window and rested on the skin surface. The bowel wall is opened via a transverse incision closer to the distal limb (Figure 7-12). The mucosal edges are everted using a series of 3-0 absorbable sutures in a rosebud type fashion (Figure 7-13) and the ostomy is completed (Figure 7-14).

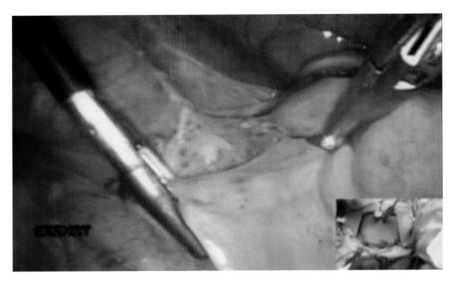

Figure 7-10 ▪ The small bowel is mobilized by division of peritoneal attachments in the region of the ileocolic junction using the bipolar vessel sealing device.

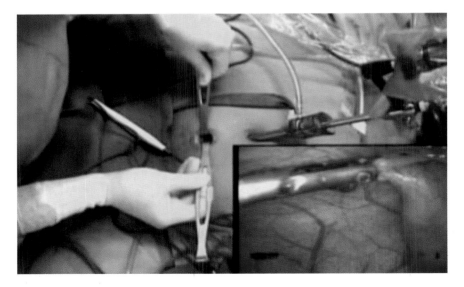

Figure 7-11 ▪ Creation of the abdominal wall defect (stoma site).

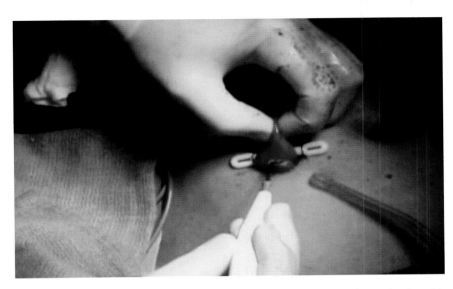

Figure 7-12 ▪ The loop of ileum is brought up through the stoma site, a plastic rod is placed through and mesenteric defect, and the bowel wall is opened via a transverse incision.

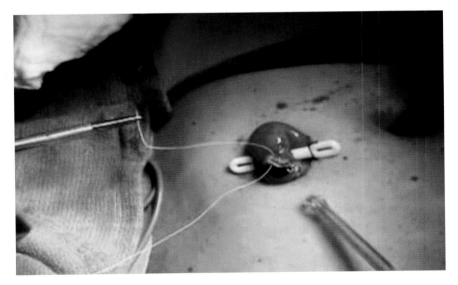

Figure 7-13 ▪ The mucosal edges are everted using a series of 3-0 absorbable sutures in a rosebud-type fashion.

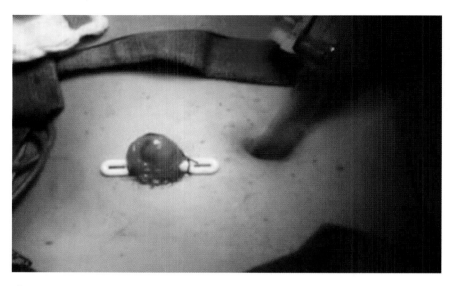

Figure 7-14 ▪ A matured loop ileostomy.

Right hemicolectomy

Senagore et al.[29] examined results of 70 laparoscopic right hemicolectomies using a standardized technique. A summary of the described technique is outlined below:

1. Open insertion of the umbilical port.
2. Placement of three additional ports.
3. Elevation of the right colic pedicle and transection of the vessels at their origin (in gynecologic oncology patients where full mesenteric resection and lymph node resection is not necessary, the vessels may be taken closer to the bowel).
4. Elevation of right colon and transverse colon off the retroperitoneum.
5. Entrance of the lesser sac with division of the gastrocolic ligament.
6. Division of the lateral peritoneal reflection.
7. Exteriorization of the specimen through a wound protector.
8. Extracorporeal division and anastomosis.

We prefer a similar "medial-to-lateral" approach in our colonic resections. In this fashion, the vascular pedicles are identified early (Figure 7-15) and separated from vital structures such as the duodenum (Figure 7-16) before mobilization of the lateral peritoneal attachments. The vessels are transected at their origin allowing for complete cytoreduction

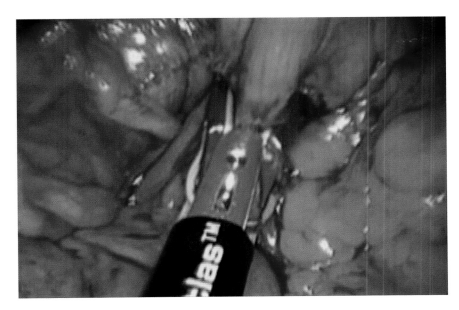

Figure 7-15 ■ The right colic and ileo-colic vessels are identified and transected using the bipolar vessel sealing device.

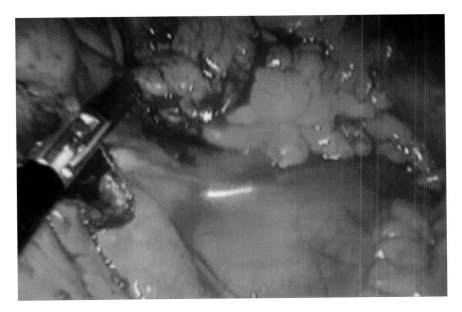

Figure 7-16 ■ As the right colon is mobilized care is taken to avoid injury to the duodenum.

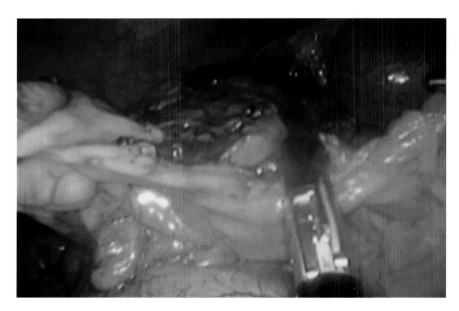

Figure 7-17 ▪ The gastrocolic ligament is divided and allows entry into the lesser sac.

and lymph node harvest if needed. Because the bowel remains tethered to the lateral abdominal wall, this acts as a source of tension allowing for easier mobilization. Once the vessels have been transected, the lesser sac is entered by dividing the gastrocolic liagament (Figure 7-17) and the hepatocolic ligament is also divided (Figure 7-18). The lateral attachments can be freed and the bowel exteriorized (Figure 7-19). While this is our preferred technique, a lateral to medial approach as is equally effective based on surgeon expertise and preference. Although no definitive studies have been published comparing laparoscopic bowel resection versus open bowel resection in the management of gynecologic cancers, extrapolating from the colorectal surgery literature suggests that outcomes would be equivalent.[30]

Left hemicolectomy

We traditionally use a medial to lateral technique for resection of the sigmoid and rectum. A hand assist device can be helpful in these procedures and is placed through a lower midline or "mini" Pfannensteil incision made slightly smaller (measured in centimeters) in size than the individuals glove size (Figure 7-20). Manual retraction of the colon allows for

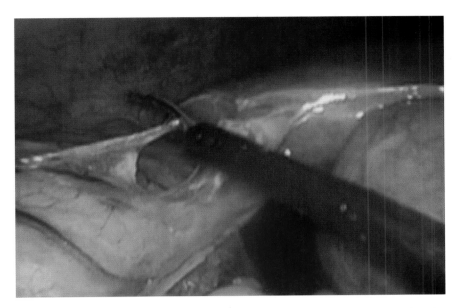

Figure 7-18 ▪ The hepatocolic ligament is divided using either unipolar or bipolar cautery.

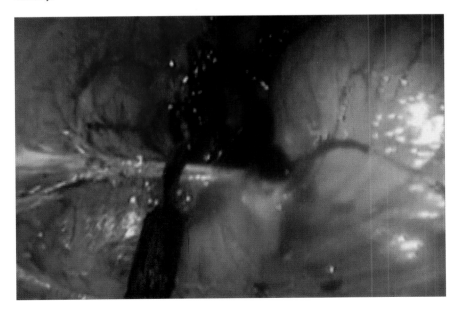

Figure 7-19 ▪ Division of lateral attachments is performed allowing full mobilization of the right colon. The bowel is then exteriorized, and an extracorporeal resection and anastomosis performed.

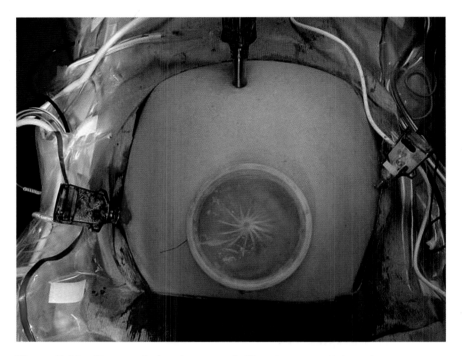

Figure 7-20 ▪ The use of a hand-port can facilitate laparoscopic bowel surgery.

easier mobilization with blunt dissection and can allow for rapid control in the presence of heavy bleeding.

In most instances this procedure is performed in conjunction with other gynecologic oncology-related procedures, and therefore both the left and right pelvic sidewalls are routinely opened and the pararectal spaces are developed allowing for identification of both ureters prior to proceeding the colon resection. This dissection is carried superiorly to the level of the common iliac vessels to allow further mobilization of the bowel (Figure 7-21). At a minimum, identification of the left ureter is mandatory prior transection of the sigmoid and superior rectal vessels. For routine sigmoid resection, it is not our preference to place ureteral stents.

Lateral peritoneal attachments can be divided using the electrocautery device after mobilization by finger dissection (Figure 7-22). The dissection is carried proximally with mobilization of the splenic flexure and division of the gastrocolic ligaments. This dissection can be technically challenging making the left hemicolectomy a procedure for more experienced laparoscopists.

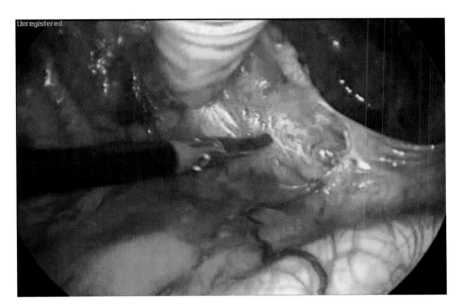

Figure 7-21 ■ We routinely develop both pararectal spaces and identify both ureters during mobilization and division of bowel mesentery. The dissection is carried superiorly to the common iliac vessels as shown here.

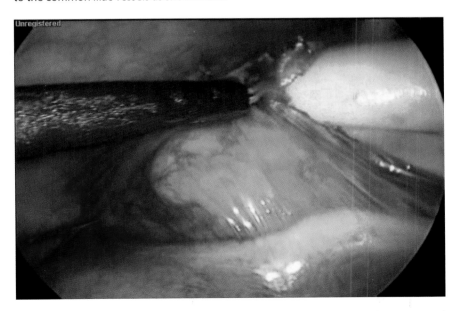

Figure 7-22 ■ The sigmoid colon is mobilized proximally with finger dissection and attachments are divided with the electrocautery.

Unlike a right hemicolectomy, the colorectal anastomosis during sigmoid resection is performed intracorporeally. After complete mobilization and division of the vessels (Figure 7-23), the bowel wall is skeletonized circumferentially and transected intracorporeally with the endostapler (Figure 7-24). The distal limb is externalized through the hand port (Figure 7-25) or with a wound protector, and the proximal margin stapled (or divided) extracorporeally. An EEA anvil placed in the proximal limb and secured down using a purse string suture (Figure 7-26). The EEA stapling device is then placed into the anus and brought up the rectosigmoid colon and the spike is deployed either through the staple line or anteriorly avoiding the mesentery (Figure 7-27). The anvil is attached and the bowel limbs are reapproximated. An intracorporeal anastomosis is then performed firing the EEA stapling device (Figure 7-28) and the anastomosis line is visualized with a sigmoidoscope and is tested for leaks with air (bubble test) and/or diluted betadine (Figure 7-29). The "donuts" in the EEA stapling device are inspected and any defects should raise suspicion about the possibility of an incomplete anastomosis.

In most colon resections, the colon becomes a midline structure and can be removed through a small periumbilical or infraumbilical incision in the midline. Small bowel resection rarely requires much mobilization

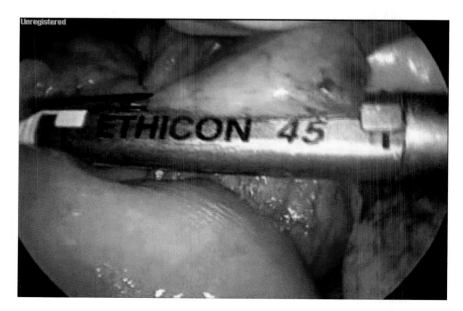

Figure 7-23 ▪ The mesentery is transected using the endoscopic gastrointestinal stapler.

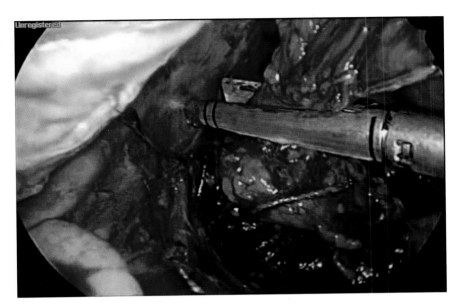

Figure 7-24 ■ The sigmoid colon is divided using the endoscopic gastrointestinal stapling device.

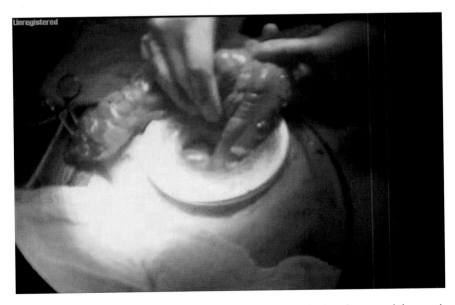

Figure 7-25 ■ The sigmoid colon is exteriorized through the hand-port and the proximal diseased segment is divided extracorporeally using the stapling device and removed from the field.

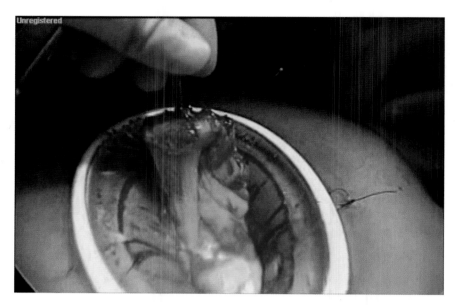

Figure 7-26 ▪ The anvil from the appropriately sized EEA stapling device is placed into the proximal colon and secured in place with a purse-string suture.

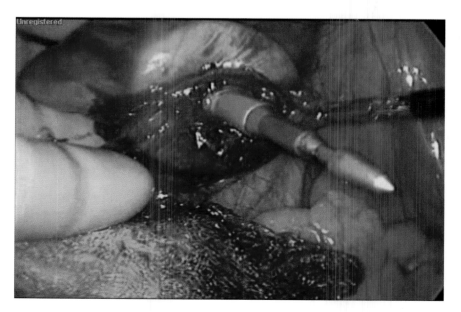

Figure 7-27 ▪ The stapler is placed into the rectal stump and the spike is deployed penetrating the bowel wall.

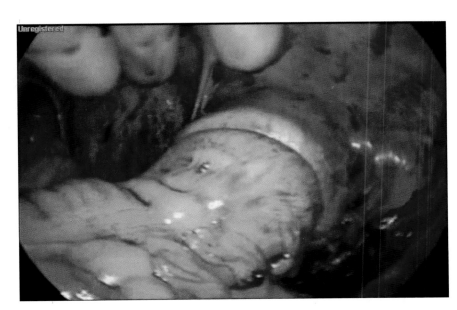

Figure 7-28 ■ The proximal and distal bowel limbs are approximated and the EEA stapling device is fired. The "donuts" are removed and checked for defects.

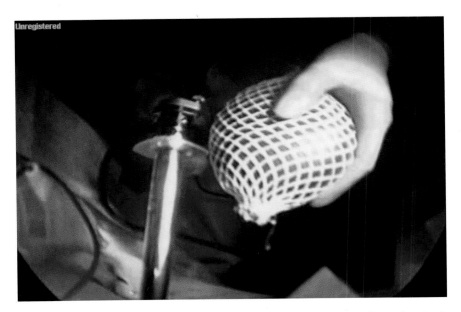

Figure 7-29 ■ The pelvis is filled with fluid and a sigmoidoscopy is performed to check for leaks (bubble test) and visualize the anastomosis.

and once the area of disease is identified, the loop of intestine can be brought out extracorporeally for resection and anastomosis. Although a sign of a skilled laparoscopist, there is little advantage to the intracorporeal anastomosis as in most instances the bowel must be removed through and abdominal incision, which always allows for the extracorporeal anastomosis.

Complications

Complications of laparoscopic bowel surgery can be grouped into three general categories. The first category includes complications that are associated with bowel surgery and are the same as those associated with traditional open bowel surgery. The second category includes complications related to major intraoperative and postoperative morbidity and are listed as category 2 complications. The final category includes complications unique to laparoscopic bowel surgery and are listed as category 3 complications.

Complications of bowel surgery in the gynecologic oncology population have been well described.[1–3,9] In previously irradiated patients undergoing low rectal resection and anastomosis at the time of pelvic exenteration, the length of the rectal stump was found to be associated with likelihood of complete healing.[9] Specifically, a rectal stump length of 6 cm or greater was associated with an 85% complete healing rate compared to 43% of patients with a rectal stump length of less than 6 cm.[9] Interestingly, one institutional review reported a concerning rate of local recurrent cancer in patients undergoing low rectal anastomosis at the time of pelvic exenteration for recurrent pelvic cancers.[8] There is a paucity of literature regarding laparoscopic or laparoscopic-assisted pelvic exenteration; however, one study reported three of five patients remaining free of disease with a mean follow-up of 10 months.[7]

One complication unique to laparoscopic surgery (compared to traditional open surgery) in patients with gynecologic cancers is the development of port site metastases. The incidence of port site metastases in patients with gynecologic malignancies undergoing laparoscopic surgery is less than 2.5%.[31] Patients with recurrent ovarian or primary peritoneal cancer undergoing laparoscopy in the presence of ascites appear to be at the highest risk for the subsequent development of port site metastases.[31] Patients with advanced or recurrent disease with progression of carcinomatosis and synchronous metastases to other sites are also considered to have a significant risk for developing port site metastases.[32] Although clinically important, the overall risk of port site metastases is low and therefore this potential risk should not be used as an argument against performing laparoscopy in patients with gynecologic malignancies.[32]

- Category 1 (Bowel surgery-related complications)
  - Bowel obstruction[1-3]
  - Ileus[2,3]
  - Bowel stricture[1,9]
  - Anastomosis leak/breakdown[1,2,4,9,14]
  - Fistula[1-3]
  - Chronic diarrhea[1]
  - Tenesmus[1]
  - Fecal incontinence[1]
  - Intra-abdominal infection/abscess[2-4,14]
  - Short bowel syndrome
  - Blind loop and/or blind pouch syndrome
  - Hernia (peristomal)[3]
- Category 2 (Major intraoperative and postoperative complications)
  - Incorrect positioning-related neuropathy[33]
  - Perioperative febrile morbidity[1,2]
  - Intraoperative complications including hemorrhage and/or transfusion, enterotomies, cystotomy, and ureteral injuries[1,2,14]
  - Wound breakdown/infection[1-3]
  - Thromboembolic events[1,4]
- Category 3 (Laparoscopic-specific complications)
  - Port site metastases[31,32]
  - Subcutaneous emphysema
  - Port-placement related vascular injury (i.e., inferior epigastric injury or injury to retroperitoneal vessels)

In the colorectal literature, the incidence of most major complications, such as anastomotic leak, sepsis, cardiac complication, respiratory complication, and venous thromboembolism have been shown to be equal for laparoscopic bowel resection versus open resection. In addition, laparoscopic bowel procedures have been associated with longer operating times, but lower rates of wound infection and bleeding-related complications.[30]

Results

The choice of whether to perform a hand-sewn anastomosis, stapled anastomosis, or combination of hand-sewn and stapled anastomosis is dependent several factors including surgeon preference, available equipment, and the specific characteristics related to the case. Importantly, studies have now shown that hand-sewn and stapled anastomosis are equivalent in terms of outcomes and that there is no difference in complication rates between single layer continuous polypropylene suture technique, double-layered suture technique (chromic running inner layer and silk interrupted outer layer), and stapled (gastrointestinal anastomosis stapling device) anastomosis.[34] Therefore, emphasis is placed on adhering to the traditional principles of bowel surgery (inverting mucosal edges, water tight anastomosis), rather than the anastomosis technique chosen.

Since there are no major publications addressing the outcome of laparoscopic bowel resection for gynecologic malignancy, we have extrapolated from the colorectal cancer literature. With intracorporeal transection of the mesenteric vessels, it has been proven repeatedly that an oncologically sound operation can be performed using minimally invasive techniques. The number of lymph nodes harvested in laparoscopic specimens compared to open specimens is equivalent; 11.8 ± 7.4 versus 12.2 ± 7.8.[35]

Outcomes between open resection and laparoscopic resection have been compared by length of operation, operating room and hospital expenses, postoperative pain control, and finally survival outcome. Four major randomized trials have been performed in North America and Europe to evaluate these outcomes and are referred to as the Barcelona,[36] Clinical Outcomes of Surgical Therapy (COST),[37] Conventional Versus Laparoscopic-Assisted Surgery in Patients with Colorectal Cancer (CLASSIC),[38] and Colon Cancer Laparoscopic or Open Resection (COLOR)[39] trials.

In 2002, Lacy et al.[36] provided the first survival data in a randomized trial comparing laparoscopic colectomy for cancer with open techniques. Surprisingly, this group described a significant survival advantage for patients with stage III colon cancer undergoing laparoscopic colectomy. However, early criticisms focused on the small number of patients enrolled in each arm (approximately 100 patients), the fact that all surgeries were performed by only one group of skilled laparoscopic surgeons, and that adjuvant therapy was not standardized between the two groups.

In 1994, the COST Study Group[37] initiated a multicenter randomized trial in the United States to evaluate laparoscopic colectomy for colon cancer. Unlike the Barcelona trial, COST was performed at 48 institutions by 66 surgeons. Each surgeon had performed more than 20 laparoscopic colectomies and had submitted a video for evaluation. In all, 863 patients were enrolled in this noninferiority trial. With median follow-up of 4.4 years, the data was presented in 2004. Importantly, a 21% conversion rate to open surgery was accepted reported, and the time to recurrence and overall survival was proven equivalent between the two techniques.

Similar results have been confirmed by two additional randomized trials in Europe, the COLOR and CLASSIC trials; however, survival outcomes have been limited to 3-year follow-up thus far. Regardless, it has been repeatedly proven that laparoscopic colectomy for colon cancer has at least equivalent survival compared to open techniques.[35,40]

There are many differences between colorectal cancer and gynecologic malignancies including patterns of disease spread, and response to adjuvant therapies. None of the above colorectal trials included metastatic colon cancer patients and therefore, patients with advanced peritoneal spread, or spread to the ovaries were excluded. By definition, bowel surgery for advanced gynecologic cancer would include peritoneal spread to these structures. Therefore, although the colorectal data provide reassurance to the gynecologic oncologist, further studies are needed to confirm these findings in the gynecologic oncology patient population.

In summary, there is a paucity of data regarding laparoscopic bowel resection for gynecologic malignancies. The majority of our understanding in this field has been extrapolated from the colorectal literature for laparoscopic colectomy in the treatment of colorectal cancer. Multiple randomized studies have demonstrated equivalent resections, morbidity and mortality for laparoscopic colectomy versus open colectomy in the colorectal literature.[40] In general, the advantages of laparoscopy including smaller incisions, less narcotic requirements, shorter hospital stays, an overall quicker recovery period and a shorter interval to adjuvant therapy hold true for patients undergoing laparoscopic bowel surgery. Therefore, gynecologic oncologists should consider these techniques in the selected patient undergoing bowel surgery for gynecologic malignancies.

REFERENCES

1. Hoffman MS, Lynch CM, Gleeson NC, Fiorica JV, Roberts WS, Cavanagh D. Colorectal anastomosis on a gynecologic oncology service. *Gynecol Oncol.* 1994;55:60–65.
2. Estes JM, Leath CA, Staughn JM, et al. Bowel resection at the time of primary debulking for epithelial ovarian carcinoma: Outcomes in patients treated with platinum and taxane-based chemotherapy. *J Am Coll Surg.* 2006;203:527–532.
3. Gillette-Cloven N, Burger RA, Monk BJ, et al. Bowel resection at the time of primary cytoreduction for epithelial ovarian cancer. *J Am Coll Surg.* 2001;193:626–632.

4. Bristow RE, del Carmen MG, Kaufman HS, Montz FJ. Radical oophorectomy with primary stapled colorectal anastomosis for resection of locally advanced epithelial ovarian cancer. *J Am Coll Surg*. 2003;197:565-574.

5. Chi DS, McCaughty K, Diaz JP, et al. Guidelines and selection criteria for secondary cytoreductive surgery in patients with recurrent, platinum-sensitive epithelial ovarian carcinoma. *Cancer*. 2006;106:1933-1939.

6. Salani R, Santillan A, Zahurak ML, et al. Secondary cytoreductive surgery for localized recurrent epithelial ovarian cancer. *Cancer*. 2007;109:685-691.

7. Ferron G, Querleu D, Martel P, Letourneur B, Soulie M. Laparoscopy-assisted vaginal pelvic exenteration. *Gynecol Oncol*. 2006;100:551-555.

8. Goldberg GL, Sukumvanich P, Einstein MH, Smith HO, Anderson PS, Fields AL. Total pelvic exenteration: The Albert Einstein College of Medicine/Montifiore Medical Center Experience (1987 to 2003). *Gynecol Oncol*. 2006;101:261-268.

9. Hatch KD, Shingleton HM, Potter ME, Baker VV. Low rectal resection and anastomosis at the time of pelvic exenteration. *Gynecol Oncol*. 1988;31:262-267.

10. Barakat RR, Goldman NA, Patel DA, Venkatraman ES, Curtin JP. Pelvic exenteration for recurrent endometrial cancer. *Gynecol Oncol*. 1999;75:99-102.

11. Awtrey CS, Cadungog MG, Leitao MM, et al. Surgical resection of recurrent endometrial carcinoma. *Gynecol Oncol*. 2006;102:480-488.

12. Bristow RE, Santillan A, Zahurak ML, Gardner GJ, Giuntoli RL, Armstrong DK. Salvage cytoreductive surgery for recurrent endometrial cancer. *Gynecol Oncol*. 2006;103:281-287.

13. Giuntoli RL, Garrett-Mayer E, Bristow RE, Gostout BS. Secondary cytoreduction in the management of recurrent leiomyosarcoma. *Gynecol Oncol*. 2007. doi:10.1016/j.ygyno.2007.02.031.

14. Duepree HJ, Senagore AJ, Delaney CP, Marcello PW, Brady KM, Falcone T. Laparoscopic resection of deep pelvic endometriosis with rectosigmoid involvement. *J Am Coll Surg*. 2002;195:754-758.

15. Lewis LA, Nezhat C. Laparoscopic treatment of bowel endometriosis. *Surg Technol Int*. 2007;16:137-141.

16. Nezhat C, Nezhat F, Pennington E. Laparoscopic treatment of infiltrative rectosigmoid colon and rectovaginal septum endometriosis by the technique of videolaserlaparoscopy and the CO_2 laser. *Br J Obstet Gynaecol*. 1992;99:664-667.

17. Nezhat C, Nezhat F, Pennington E. Laparoscopic proctectomy for infiltrating endometriosis of the rectum. *Fertil Steril*. 1992;57:1129-1132.

18. Maxwell GL, Synan I, Dodge R, Carroll B, Clarke-Pearson DL. Pneumatic compression versus low molecular weight heparin in gynecologic oncology surgery: A randomized trial. *Obstet Gynecol*. 2001;98:989-995.

19. Clarke-Pearson DL, Dodge RK, Synan I, McClelland RC, Maxwell GL. Venous thromboembolism prophylaxis: Patients at high risk to fail intermittent pneumatic compression. *Obstet Gynecol*. 2003;101:157-163.

20. Nezhat C, Nezhat F, Ambroze W, Pennington E. Laparoscopic repair of small bowel and colon. *Surg Endoscopy*. 1993;7:88-89.

21. Curran TJ, Borzotta AP. Complications of primary repair of colon injury: Literature review of 2964 cases. *Am J Surg*. 1999;177:42–47.

22. Conrad JK, Ferry KM, Foreman ML, et al. Changing management trends in penetrating colon trauma. *Dis Colon Rectum*. 2000;43:466–471.

23. Bucher P, Mermillod B, Gervas P, et al. Mechanical bowel preparation for elective colorectal surgery: A meta-analysis. *Arch Surg*. 2004;139:1359–1364.

24. Bucher P, Gervas P, Soravia C, et al. Randomized clinical trial of mechanical bowel preparation versus no preparation before elective left-sided colorectal surgery. *Br J Surg*. 2005;48:1509–1516.

25. Muzii L, Bellati F, Zullo MA, et al. Mechanical bowel preparation before gynecologic laparoscopy: A randomized, single-blind, controlled trial. *Fertil Steril*. 2006;85:689–693.

26. Nelson R, Edwards S, Tse B. Prophylactic nasogastric decompression after abdominal surgery (review). *Cochrane Rev*. 2007;2:1–31.

27. Bradshaw BG, Liu SS, Thirlby RC. Standardized perioperative care protocols and reduced length of stay after colon surgery. *J Am Coll Surg*. 1998;186:501–506.

28. Basse L, Hjort Jakobsen D, Billesbolle P, Werner M, Kehlet H. A clinical pathway to accelerate recovery after colonic resection. *Ann Surg*. 2000;232:51–57.

29. Senagore AJ, Delaney CP, Brady KM, Fazio VW. Standardized approach to laparoscopic right colectomy: Outcomes in 70 consecutive cases. *J Am Coll Surg*. 2004;199:675–679.

30. Noel JK, Fahrback K, Estok R, et al. Minimally invasive colorectal resection outcomes: Short-term comparison with open procedures. *J Am Coll Surg*. 2007;204:291–307.

31. Nagarsheth NP, Rahaman J, Cohen CJ, Gretz H, Nezhat F. The incidence of port-site metastases in gynecologic cancers. *JSLS*. 2004;8:133–139.

32. Abu-Rustum NR, Rhee Eh, Chi DS, Sonoda Y, Gemignani M, Barakat RR. Subcutaneous tumor implantation after laparoscopic procedures in women with malignant disease. *Obstet Gynecol*. 2004;103:480–487.

33. Irvin W, Andersen W, Taylor P, Rice L. Minimizing the risk of neurologic injury in gynecologic surgery. *Obstet Gyneol*. 2004;103:374–382.

34. Ceraldi CM, Rypins EB, Monahan M, Chang B, Sarfeh IJ. Comparison of continuous single layer polypropylene anastomosis with double layer and stapled anastomoses in elective colon resections. *Am Surg*. 1993;59:168–171.

35. Transatlantic Laparoscopically Assisted vs. Open Colectomy Trials Study Group. Laparoscopically assisted vs. open colectomy for colon cancer. A meta-analysis. *Arch Surg*. 2007;142:298–303.

36. Lacy AM, Garcia-Valdecasas JC, Delgado S, et al. Laparoscopy-assised colectomy versus open colectomy for treatment of non-metastatic colon cancer: A randomised trial. *Lancet*. 2002;359:2224–2229.

37. Clinical Outcomes of Surgical Therapy (COST) Study Group. A comparison of laparoscopically assisted and open colectomy for colon cancer. *N Engl J Med*. 2004;350:2050–2059.

38. Guillou PJ, Quirke P, Thorpe H, Walker J, et al. Short-term endpoints of conventional versus laparoscopic-assisted surgery in patients with colorectal cancer (MRC CLASICC Trial): Multicenter, randomised controlled trial. *Lancet.* 2005;365:1718–1726.

39. The Colon cancer Laparoscopic or Open Resection Study Group. Laparoscopic surgery versus open surgery for colon cancer: Short-term outcomes of a randomised trial. *Lancet Oncol.* 2005;6:477–484.

40. Jackson TD, Kaplan GG, Arena G, et al. Laparoscopic versus open resection for colorectal cancer: A meta-analysis of oncologic outcomes. *J Am Coll Surg.* 2007;204:439–446.

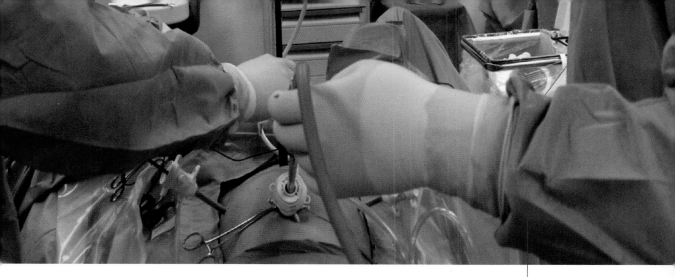

RADICAL VAGINAL TRACHELECTOMY | 8

Mario E. Beiner and Allan L. Covens

▌INTRODUCTION

Radical vaginal trachelectomy (RVT) with laparoscopic pelvic lymphadenectomy is a fertility-preserving procedure that has recently gained worldwide acceptance as an acceptable method of surgically treating small invasive cancers of the cervix. The RVT was pioneered by Dargent et al.[1] in the late 1980s; the authors reported their first series of cases at the annual meeting of the Society of Gynecologic Oncologists in 1994. The procedure involves removing most, if not all, of the cervix, its contiguous parametrium, and vaginal cuff. In addition a laparoscopic pelvic lymphadenectomy is usually performed also. Since that original description, over 500 cases utilizing this technique have been reported in the literature, with over 100 live births reported following this procedure.[2]

INDICATIONS

- Desire to preserve fertility.
- Tumor size less or equal to 2 cm.
- FIGO stage IA1 with lymph vascular space invasion (LVSI), stage IA2, stage IB1.
- Squamous histology or adenocarcinoma.

CONTRAINDICATIONS

- Involvement of the upper endocervical canal.
- FIGO stage >IB1.
- Contraindications to vaginal surgery.
- Tumor >2 cm.
- Patient does not wish preservation of fertility.
- Indications on cone biopsy or MRI that adjuvant radiation therapy will be required or recommended.

EQUIPMENT

- Speculums:
  - Weighted speculum-long blade
- Retractors:
  - Breisky
  - Sims
- Clamps:
  - Lauer
  - Croback
  - Heaney or Rogers
  - Snaps
  - Needle drivers
- Forceps:
  - Mayo
  - Bonney
  - Tissue nontooth
- Suture:
  - Mersilene (BP-1 RS21)
  - Polysorb 2-0 (delayed absorbable)

- Scissor:
  - Mayo straight
  - Mayo curved
  - Metzenbaum
- Tenaculum:
  - Single tooth
- Other:
  - Vasopressin 20 units in 100 mL of IV normal saline
  - 8 FR catheter
  - Foley catheter 14 FR + urine bag
  - Knife handle
  - Cautery

SETUP AND PATIENTS POSITIONING

- The operating suite is prepared for laparoscopy and vaginal surgery.
- The patient is placed in the semidorsal lithotomy position, with a foley catheter inserted into the bladder.

TECHNIQUE

The surgical procedure generally begins with a laparoscopic pelvic lymphadenectomy or sentinel pelvic lymph node biopsy. This part of the procedure can be performed by a transperitoneal or retroperitoneal approach. Similarly, for those surgeons unskilled in laparoscopy, it is possible to perform this part of the surgery by an extraperitoneal dissection.

The RVT starts by infiltrating the vaginal mucosa around the cervix with diluted vasopressin solution. The vaginal mucosa is incised circumferentially by scalpel, leaving an adequate vaginal margin (usually 1–2 cm). The posterior cul de sac is sharply entered, and the most distal aspect of the uterosacral ligaments are isolated and divided in their mid portion.

The anterior portion of the dissection begins by sharply developing the vesicouterine space, while downward traction is placed on the specimen. The peritoneum overlying the anterior cul de sac is *not* incised. Once the vesicouterine space is developed, the paravesical space is identified by a small indentation created by retracting the vaginal cuff at 12 o'clock and 3 (or 9) o'clock positions. Using a long curved Kelly, the paravesical space is developed by tunneling in an antero-lateral direction. Cooper's ligament should be palpable anteriorly. The tissue between the paravesical and vesicouterine space is the vesicouterine ligament. A Breisky retractor is placed in the paravesical space, and the ureter can be palpated (clicked) against the retractor. The distal aspect of the left vesicouterine ligament can now be transected superiorly up to the level of the ureter. The knee of the ureter is identified by dissecting inferiorly, parallel and posteriorly to the ureter. The portions of the cardinal and uterosacral ligaments to be transected are identified.

The parametrium is clamped, divided, and ligated to obtain an adequate margin. The cervicovaginal branch of the left uterine artery is clamped, divided and ligated. By paplpating posteriorly, the cervico uterine junction can be palpated and a suitable portion of the cervix is transected from the fundus. A frozen section is performed on the superior margin of the cervix to confirm a minimum of 5 mm tumor clearance. For those patients where the margin appears to be less, further resection of the cervix/lower uterine segment is performed until the above criterion is met. A No. 8 French rubber catheter is inserted and sutured into the os of the "neocervix" to maintain patency. To prevent cervical incompetence, a Mersilene (Shirodkar) suture is placed around the lower uterine segment and tied posteriorly. Alternatively, the Shirodkar suture can be placed at a later date in late first trimester after confirming a viable pregnancy. Finally, the vaginal cuff is sutured to the most lateral portions of the "neocervix" while burying the Mersilene suture.

Laparoscopy may be performed as the final step in the procedure to assure pelvic hemostasis.

PRE– AND POSTSURGERY MANAGEMENT

Presurgery

The patient is admitted to hospital on the same day of surgery, after 24 hours of clear fluid diet and fasting from midnight.

Postsurgery

The patient is discharged on the same day with a Foley catheter draining the bladder. The catheter is removed after 3 to 5 days, and a postvoid residual (<100 cc) performed to confirm normal bladder function. The rubber catheter that was placed in the cervical os is removed after 3 weeks.

Follow-up is every 3 months for 2 years, then every 6 months for 3 years, and then yearly. Each visit entails Pap smear and colposcopy in addition to the usual history and physical examination.

During pregnancy, these patients should be followed by an obstetrician, in a high risk pregnancy clinic setting, as preterm rupture of membranes is common. One to the Shirodkar suture, caesarean section is required for delivery.

Adjuvant therapy should be offered in cases of metastasis to LN, parametrial involvement, positive margins, or in patients with high-risk features (deep invasion, vascular space involvement).

COMPLICATIONS

Intraoperative complications

- Bladder, ureteral, bowel injury.
- Vascular (epigastric, iliacs, obturator), nerve (genitofemoral, obturator) injury (during lymphadenectomy).
- Bleeding (parametrium, sidewall).

Postoperative complications

- Bladder hypotonia.
- Lymphocyst, lymphedema.
- Isthmic stenosis.
- Wound infection, hernia.
- Leg weakness, numbness.

RESULTS

Seven groups have reported on their experience with RVT[3–9] and the results were summarized in a recent review[2] and in Tables 8-1 to 8-3. With a mean follow-up for the combined series of approximately 4 years, recurrences have occurred in 5% of the cases, and death caused by disease in 3% (Table 3-2). No significant differences have been detected in the

Table 8-1

Table 8-1 PATIENTS AND TUMOR CHARACTERISTICS

Author(s)	N	Age (y)	Stage						Size		Histology			+LVSI	+LN
			IA1	IA2	IB1	IB2	IIA	IIB	≤2 cm	≥2 cm	Squam	Adeno*	Other		
Shepherd et al.[6]	123	31	—	2 (2%)	121 (98%)	—	—	—	NR	NR	83 (68%)	36 (29%)	4 (11%)	39 (32%)	7/123 (6%)
Hertel et al.[5]	108	32	18 (17%)	21 (19%)	69 (64%)	—	—	—	108 (100%)	—	75 (69%)	33 (31%)	—	38 (35%)	4/108 (4%)
Mathevet et al.[12]	109†	32	13 (14%)	14 (14%)	56 (59%)	1 (1%)	7 (7%)	5 (5%)	67 (70%)	28 (30%)	76 (80%)	19 (20%)	1	23 (24%)	8/109 (7%)
Covens[4]	93	30	39 (42%)	22 (24%)	31 (33%)	1 (1%)	—	—	85 (91%)	8 (9%)	40 (43%)	50 (54%)	3 (3%)	31 (33%)	2/93 (2%)
Plante et al.[8]	82	31	4 (5%)	24 (30%)	51 (61%)	—	3 (4%)	—	72 (90%)	10 (10%)	49 (60%)	32 (39%)	1 (1%)	17 (21%)	5/82 (6%)
Burnett et al.[9]	21	30	—	1 (5%)	20 (95%)	—	—	—	Mean size 1.1 cm (0.3–3 cm)		12 (57%)	9 (43%)	—	3 (14%)	1/21 (5%)
Schlearth et al.[7]	12‡	31	—	8 (80%)	2 (20%)	—	—	—	10 (83%)	2 (17%)	4 (40%)	6 (60%)	—	1 (10%)	0/12 (0%)
Total	548	31	74 (14%)	92 (17%)	350 (66%)	2 (0.5%)	10 (1.5%)	5 (1%)	342/389 (88%)	48/389 (12%)	339 (64%)	185 (34%)	9 (2%)	152 (28%)	27/548 (5%)

* Including adenosquamous.
† Missing information on additional 13 patients that trachelectomy was abandoned.
‡ Missing information on additional two patients that underwent completion radical hysterectomy.

Table 8-2   **RECURRENCE DATA**

Author(s)	N	LN Metastasis +	LN Metastasis −	Histology Adeno*	Histology Squam	Tumor Size >2 cm	Tumor Size <2 cm	LVSI +	LVSI −	Time to Recurrence (mo)	Median F/U (mo)	Death
Shepherd et al.[6]	5/123 (4%)	2/7 (28%)	3/116 (3%)	NR	NR	NR	NR	1/39 (2%)	4/84 (5%)	34 (15–84)	45 (1–120)	4
Hertel et al.[5]	4/108 (4%)	0/4 (0%)	4/104 (4%)	3/33 (9%)	1/75 (1%)	1/1 (100%)	0/107 (0%)	NR	NR	14 (3–34)	29 (1–128)	2
Mathevet et al.[12]	4/108‡ (4%)	NR	NR	1/19 (5%)	3/76 (4%)	4/28 (14%)	0/68 (0%)	3/23 (13%)	1/72 (1%)	34 (7–93)	76 (4–176)	3
Covens[4]	7/93 (7%)	1/2 (50%)	6/92 (6%)	3/44 (7%)	4/42 (9%)	1/8 (12%)	6/85 (70%)	6/31 (19%)	1/62 (0%)	NR	30 (1–103)	4
Plante et al.[8]	6/82 (7%)	1/5 (20%)	5/77 (6%)	†1/30 (3%)	†2/42 (5%)	†2/8 (25%)	†1/64 (1%)	NR	NR	25 (9–60)	60 (6–156)	4
Burnett et al.[9]	2/21 (10%)	0/1	2/20	NR	NR	NR	NR	2/3	0/18	—	31 (8–81)	0
Schlearth et al.[7]	†0/12 (0%)	0/0	0/12	0/6	0/4	0/2	0/10	0/1	0/11	—	48 (28–84)	0
Total	26/548 (5.1%)	4/19 (21%)	18/421 (5%)	8/141 (6%)	10/251 (4%)	8/47 (17%)	7/334 (2%)	12/97 (12%)	6/247 (2%)	27 (3–93)	47 (1–176)	17/548 (3.1%)

* Including adenosquamous.
† Missing information on other recurrences.
‡ Missing information on 13 abandoned cases.
NR, not reported.

Table 8-3 OBSTETRICAL OUTCOMES OF PATIENTS THAT UNDERWENT TRACHELECTOMY

Authors	N	Women Attempting Pregnancy	Women Achieving Pregnancy	Number of Pregnancies	SA	EUP	TOP	Second Trimester Loss	Ongoing	Third Trimester Deliveries			Total Live Births
										24–32 wk	33–36 wk	≥37 wk	
Shepherd et al.[6]	112	63	26 (41%)	55	14 (25%)	1 (2%)	2 (4%)	7 (13%)	3 (5%)	7 (13%)	13 (24%)	8 (14%)	28
Herrel et al.[5]	100	NR	NR	18	1 (5%)	—	2 (11%)	—	3 (16%)	NR			12
Mathevet et al.[12]	95	42	33 (79%)	56	9 (16%)	2 (4%)	3 (5%)	8 (14%)	—		5 (9%)	29 (52%)	34
Bernardini et al.[13]	80	39	18 (46%)	22	3 (14%)	—	—	1 (4%)	—	3* (14%)	3 (14%)	12 (54%)	19
Plante et al.[11]	72	NR	31	50	8 (16%)	—	2 (4%)	2 (4%)	2 (4%)	3 (6%)	5 (10%)	28 (56%)	36
Burnett et al.[9]	18	4	3 (75%)	3	—	—	—	1 (33%)	—	1* (34%)	—	1 (33%)	3
Schlearth et al.[7]	10	NR	4	4	—	—	—	2 (50%)	—	1 (25%)	—	1 (25%)	2
Total	487	—	—	208	17%	1%	4%	10%	4%	—	—	—	134 (64%)

* Includes twins.

SA, spontaneous abortions; EUP, extra uterine pregnancy; TOP, termination of pregnancy; NR, not reported.

recurrence rates from these pooled series of patients compared to historical controls. Nearly 40% of recurrences have been to the parametrium/pelvic sidewall, raising the possibility of insufficient parametrial excision. Approximately 25% of the recurrences were to lymph nodes either pelvic, paraaortic or supraclavicular. The technique of sentinel node mapping may help localize aberrant nodal metastasis spread, and/or identify micrometastases which have been missed with conventional histopathologic processing and may explain some nodal recurrences in the face of a negative pelvic lymphadenectomy. Four cases of central recurrence in the residual cervix or uterus were reported by two centers included in this review.[5-6]

From analyzing the reports of the seven groups it appears that the recurrence rate is higher among cases with a lesion size >2 cm. Although not clearly associated with a higher risk recurrence, the presence of LVSI is another high-risk feature to consider.

Of the reported pregnancy outcomes (Table 8-3), there have been 208 pregnancies, resulting in 134 (64%) live births, following RVT. In the reports that included information on the number of women attempting pregnancy, between 41% and 79% of patients were successful. The rate of first trimester miscarriage was 18%, similar to the general population. Term delivery ($\geq$37 wk) was reached in 38% of all pregnancies. The most common complication following this procedure is second trimester loss and premature delivery. The rate of second trimester loss was 10% and preterm delivery (<37 wk) was observed in 20% of the pregnancies. Infertility has been described in 25% to 30% of the patients attempting to conceive.[10-11] Subsequently, intrauterine insemination, ovarian stimulation, and in vitro fertilization have been successfully utilized in these patients.

In summary, RVT appears to be a safe procedure with recurrence rates of approximately 5%. With an expected term delivery rate greater than 50%, RVT seems to be the procedure of choice for women with small early stage cervical cancers wishing to preserve their fertility.

REFERENCES

1. Dargent D, Brun JL, Roy M, Remy I. Pregnancies following radical trachelectomy for invasive cervical cancer. *Gynecol Oncol.* 1994;52(1):105.
2. Beiner ME, Covens A. Surgery insight: Radical vaginal trachelectomy as a method of fertility preservation for cervical cancer. *Nat Clin Pract Oncol.* 2007;4(6):353–361.

3. Marchiole P, Marchiole P, Benchaib M, Buenerd A, Lazlo E, Dargent D, Mathevet P. Oncological safety of laparoscopic-assisted vaginal radical trachelectomy (LARVT or Dargent's operation): A comparative study with laparoscopic-assisted vaginal radical hysterectomy (LARVH). *Gynecol Oncol.* 2007;106(1):132–141.

4. Covens A. Preserving fertility in early cervical Ca with radical trachelectomy. *Contemporary Ob Gyn.* 2003;2:46–66.

5. Hertel H, Köhler C, Grund D, et al. Radical vaginal trachelectomy (RVT) combined with laparoscopic pelvic lymphadenectomy: Prospective multicenter study of 100 patients with early cervical cancer. *Gynecol Oncol.* 2006;103(2):506–511.

6. Shepherd JH, Spencer C, Herod J, Ind TE. Radical vaginal trachelectomy as a fertility-sparing procedure in women with early-stage cervical cancer-cumulative pregnancy rate in a series of 123 women. *BJOG.* 2006;113(6):719–724.

7. Schlaerth JB, Spirtos NM, Schlaerth AC. Radical trachelectomy and pelvic lymphadenectomy with uterine preservation in the treatment of cervical cancer. *Am J Obstet Gynecol.* 2003;188(1):29–34.

8. Plante M, Renaud MC, François H, Roy M. Vaginal radical trachelectomy: An oncologically safe fertility-preserving surgery. An updated series of 72 cases and review of the literature. *Gynecol Oncol.* 2004;94(3):614–623.

9. Burnett AF, Roman LD, O'Meara AT, Morrow CP. Radical vaginal trachelectomy and pelvic lymphadenectomy for preservation of fertility in early cervical carcinoma. *Gynecol Oncol.* 2003;88(3):419–423.

10. Boss EA, Van Golde RJT, Beerendonk CCM, Massuger LFAG. Pregnancy after radical trachelectomy: A real option? *Gynecol Oncol.* 2005;99(3 Suppl 1):S152–S156.

11. Plante M, Renaud MC, Hoskins IA, Roy M. Vaginal radical trachelectomy: A valuable fertility-preserving option in the management of early-stage cervical cancer. A series of 50 pregnancies and review of the literature. *Gynecol Oncol.* 2005; 98(1):3–10.

12. Mathevet P, Laszlo de Kaszon E, Dargent D. Fertility preservation in early cervical cancer. *Gynecol Obstet Fertil.* 2003;31(9):706–712.

13. Bernardini M, Barrett J, Seaward G, Covens A. Pregnancy outcomes in patients after radical trachelectomy. *Am J Obstet Gynecol.* 2003;189(5):1378–1382.

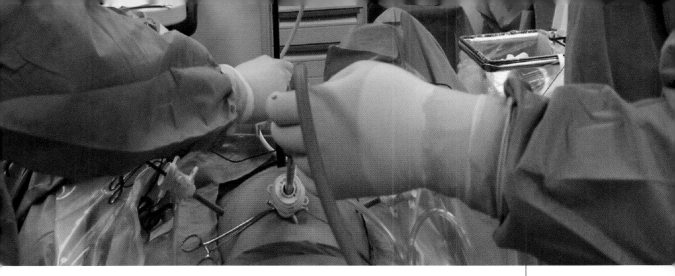

VIDEO–ASSISTED THORACOSCOPY | 9

Ram Eitan and Dennis S. Chi

INDICATIONS

Video-assisted thoracoscopic surgery (VATS) has evolved over the years from a limited procedure into an important tool for the diagnosis of many thoracic diseases and for use in a variety of intrathoracic resections. Many procedures that once required thoracotomy are now being performed using VATS, subsequently reducing surgical trauma, decreasing postoperative pain, and preserving pulmonary function.[1,2] VATS is widely used in the diagnosis and management of various thoracic diseases, such as in the staging of lung cancer, in the performance of lobectomies and wedge resections, in the diagnosis and management of pleural pathologies, and in many other pathologic situations involving the chest. The most common indications for VATS are in the diagnosis and evaluation of thoracic disease—pleural effusions of unknown etiology, evaluation of interstitial lung disease, and definitive diagnosis of indeterminate lung nodules.

Our interest in VATS arises from the gaining acceptance of this modality in certain clinical situations in the field of gynecologic oncology, in which VATS may play diagnostic and therapeutic roles.[3]

At present, stage IV disease is diagnosed in approximately 10% of patients with epithelial ovarian cancer.[4] In these advanced cases, a malignant pleural effusion is frequently found, but the pleural spaces and lung parenchyma may be involved to different degrees. Fallopian tube, primary peritoneal, and, in rare cases, endometrial carcinomas may also present with pleural effusions and pleural-based disease.

A pleural effusion can be accompanied by undiagnosed macroscopic pleural-based disease; the presence of macroscopic intrathoracic disease may alter patient management, particularly, if unresectable; larger than 1- to 2-cm intrathoracic tumor deposits would leave the patient with suboptimal residual disease at the conclusion of maximum intra-abdominal cytoreduction.

In addition, VATS may assist the surgeon in the assessment of diaphragmatic disease, as the extent of diaphragmatic disease may not be fully appreciated via laparotomy and dilemmas regarding whether or not to perform a full-thickness resection of the diaphragm in lieu of a diaphragm peritonectomy may arise during debulking surgery.

We usually perform VATS just before planned debulking surgery during the same operating room session, thus utilizing its complete diagnostic and therapeutic potential without delaying laparotomy. When the thoracic procedure is concluded, we then proceed with laparotomy. Indications for VATS may include the following:

1. Diagnosis of macroscopic intrathoracic malignant disease when pleural effusion is found in a patient with advanced mullerian malignancy.
2. Treatment of malignant pleural effusion.
3. Resection of intrathoracic bulky disease and/or ablation of pleural-based disease in the setting of the maximal debulking effort.
4. Assessment of full-thickness diaphragmatic involvement.

CONTRAINDICATIONS

Relative contraindications for VATS:

1. No intra-abdominal surgical effort is planned, except when treating malignant pleural effusion.
2. Ventilator dependency.

3. Noncompliant lung.
4. Severe emphysema.
5. Chest wall involvement by tumor.
6. Small thoracic cavity or significant anatomic restrictions.
7. Hemodynamic instability.
8. Coagulopathy.

PERFORMING VATS

Setup, patient positioning, and equipment

A competent anesthetic team experienced in thoracic procedures is important, as VATS cannot be performed without unilateral pulmonary atelectasis. Intubation is preferably performed with a double-lumen tube, which allows one-lung ventilation and ensures collapse of the chosen lung.

For a diagnostic procedure without a difficult resection, a single surgeon can hold the camera and possibly the biopsy forceps, and one monitor may suffice. If two surgeons are needed, two monitors are placed on either side of the patient's head, providing the best views for both members of the operating team.[2,5] The patient is placed in the lateral decubitus position as for conventional thoracotomy. To ensure maximal stretching of the intercostal spaces and to avoid obstruction to camera movement, the operating room table is slanted downward on both sides of the center so as to lower the pelvis and head.

The first trocar is meant for the camera, as in laparoscopy. A 10-mm or 5-mm trocar can be used depending on availability and operator preference. The first trocar is placed along the mid-axillary line in the sixth intercostal space. This location provides an excellent view of all pleural spaces, the lung parenchyma, and the mediastinum. The skin incision is made parallel and above the seventh rib. A small clamp is introduced through the intercostal muscles and pleura *above* the rib, taking care not to harm the intercostal blood vessels and nerve. The clamp is opened, widening the intercostal space. Some surgeons advocate the direct digital exploration of the pleural cavity beneath the incision. The first trocar is then inserted, again avoiding the blood vessels running inferior to the rib.

If pleural effusion is present, it is drained through the trocar and sent for cytology. The 10- or 5-mm camera is inserted and video-assisted exploration of the pleural cavity is performed. Operative ports may now be positioned, if needed. The operative ports are usually put along the anterior and posterior axillary line between the fourth and sixth intercostal spaces. Some surgeons advocate performing the anterior skin incision under the mammary fold to improve the cosmetic result. If malignant lesions are found, they can be biopsied or resected. Care should be taken to avoid seeding of tumor cells during extraction of tissue from the chest. A plastic endobag should be used for the larger specimens.

Pleural disease can be ablated or resected as peritoneal disease is treated in the abdomen. This can be accomplished using the argon beam coagulator and monopolar electrocautery. Loculations of pleural effusion can be entered and drained.

All of the instruments that might be needed for an emergency thoracotomy must be ready in the operating room, and the staff should be ready for a conversion, if needed.

At the end of the procedure, trocars are removed and the lung inflated. A chest drainage tube may be placed in the pleural cavity through one of the ports of entry to treat pneumothorax and drain pleural effusion in the postoperative period. All other ports are closed in layers to ensure airtight closure.

Pre- and postoperative management

Patients are followed postoperatively with daily chest radiographs to ensure that the pneumothorax is not enlarging and that the chest tube is positioned properly without kinking. In cases of malignant pleural effusions, pleurodesis can be performed with talc or doxycycline. When the pleural drainage is less than 200 to 300 cc per day, the chest tube can be removed at the bedside, making sure the incision is closed immediately after tube removal.

| COMPLICATIONS

Complications of VATS are similar to those of conventional thoracotomy, such as air leak, postoperative bleeding, wound infections, empyema, and, in rare cases, respiratory failure.[6] Some of the less common complications include pneumonia, atelectasis, arrhythmias, and deep vein thrombosis. Pulmonary edema is not reported as a VATS-specific complication but is known to be related to pneumonectomies and lobectomies. Fluid overload should be avoided, and any acute respiratory complaint in the first 24 to 48 hours postoperatively should be worked up thoroughly.

There are, however, complications related to VATS and specifically to the insertion of the thoracoscopy ports. These complications include intercostal neuritis and port site metastasis of tumor.

Port-related complications can be minimized by good surgical technique, and pain can be decreased substantially.[5] Blunt-tip ports designed for thoracoscopy should be used, and the port should be introduced without force and under control. Some surgeons advocate making the skin incision directly over the intercostal space, avoiding oblique access. Excessive spreading of intercostal tissue should be avoided.

A retrieval device will minimize the chances of port site recurrence.

RESULTS

The benefits of debulking in patients with malignant pleural effusions compared with other stage IV disease criteria have been evaluated, with mixed results. Although several retrospective reviews have demonstrated a survival benefit to optimal intra-abdominal debulking in patients with malignant pleural effusions, these patients still have decreased survival when compared with patients who have disease confined to the abdomen.[7,8]

Evaluating optimally cytoreduced stage IIIC and stage IV patients (by pleural effusion criteria), Eitan et al.[9] reported a median survival of 58 months for patients who had stage IIIC disease and 30 months for patients with stage IV disease ($p = 0.016$). While the poorer prognosis likely reflects the more aggressive and advanced nature of disease that extends extraperitoneally, the authors raise the question of whether undetected bulky residual intrathoracic disease contributes to this difference.

Chi et al.[3] initially addressed VATS as a beneficial procedure in patients with moderate to large pleural effusions, and in a follow-up study by Juretzka et al.,[10] 65% of patients had macroscopic intrathoracic disease, including 10 (83%) of 12 with positive cytology and 4 (40%) of 10 with negative cytology. More importantly, 11 (73%) of 15 patients with macroscopic intrathoracic disease had nodules greater than 1 cm. If these patients had gone on to have extensive abdominal cytoreduction, the large-volume intrathoracic disease theoretically might have negated the beneficial effects of the abdominal surgical debulking. By demonstrating unresectable macroscopic (>1 cm) disease, VATS is an important diagnostic procedure that can identify appropriate candidates for consideration of neoadjuvant chemotherapy.

VATS has shown potential to advance primary surgical approaches in ovarian cancer. Numerous studies have shown that the use of more extensive ablative techniques and radical upper abdominal procedures is often required to achieve optimal cytoreduction. In this context, diaphragmatic disease is of particular interest. VATS may be helpful in evaluating the extent of full-thickness, bulky diaphragmatic disease and can then be used to plan appropriate intra-abdominal surgical approaches.

In patients with isolated pleural-based disease, VATS may also facilitate intrathoracic cytoreduction. Eisenkop reported the outcomes of 30 patients who had undergone thoracoscopy. In this series, 33% (10 of 30 patients) of the patients had undergone pleural implant ablation and/or tumor excision, which influenced the final cytoreductive outcome.[11] Intrathoracic cytoreduction may be beneficial in select patients.

In conclusion, we believe that VATS should be incorporated into the standard management algorithm for patients with advanced ovarian cancer and moderate to large pleural effusions. Further study is necessary to evaluate the use of VATS in patients with small pleural effusions and to determine the safety and efficacy of intrathoracic cytoreduction.

REFERENCES

1. Roviaro GC, Varoli F, Vergani C, et al. State of the art in thoracoscopic surgery: A personal experience of 2000 videothoracoscopic procedures and an overview of the literature. *Surg Endosc*. 2002;16:881–892.
2. Roviaro G, Varoli F, Vergani C, et al. Video-assisted thoracoscopic major pulmonary resections: Technical aspects, personal series of 259 patients, and review of the literature. *Surg Endosc*. 2004;18:1551–1558.
3. Chi DS, Abu-Rustum NR, Sonoda Y, et al. The benefit of video-assisted thoracoscopic surgery before planned abdominal exploration in patients with suspected advanced ovarian cancer and moderate to large pleural effusions. *Gynecol Oncol*. 2004;94:307–311.
4. FIGO (International Federation of Gynecology and Obstetrics) annual report on the results of treatment in gynecological cancer. *Int J Gynaecol Obstet*. 2003; 83(Suppl 1:ix–xxii):1–229.
5. Landreneau RJ, Mack MJ, Hazelrigg SR, et al. Video-assisted thoracic surgery: Basic technical concepts and intercostal approach strategies. *Ann Thorac Surg*. 1992; 54:800–807.
6. Yim AP, Liu HP. Complications and failures of video-assisted thoracic surgery: Experience from two centers in Asia. *Ann Thorac Surg*. 1996;61:538–541.
7. Bristow RE, Montz FJ, Lagasse LD, et al. Survival impact of surgical cytoreduction in stage IV epithelial ovarian cancer. *Gynecol Oncol*. 1999;72:278–287.

8. Munkarah AR, Hallum AV III, Morris M, et al. Prognostic significance of residual disease in patients with stage IV epithelial ovarian cancer. *Gynecol Oncol.* 1997;64:13–17.

9. Eitan R, Levine DA, Abu-Rustum N, et al. The clinical significance of malignant pleural effusions in patients with optimally debulked ovarian carcinoma. *Cancer.* 2005103:1397–1401.

10. Juretzka MM, Abu-Rustum NR, Sonoda Y, et al. The impact of video-assisted thoracic surgery (VATS) in patients with suspected advanced ovarian malignancies and pleural effusions. *Gynecol Oncol.* 2007;104:670–674.

11. Eisenkop SM. Thoracoscopy for the management of advanced epithelial ovarian cancer—a preliminary report. *Gynecol Oncol.* 2002;84:315–320.

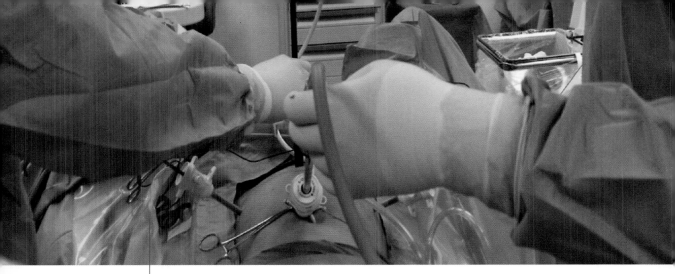

10 LAPAROSCOPIC URETERIC REIMPLANTATION AND CYSTOTOMY REPAIR

Katherine Moore and Walid Farhat

INTRODUCTION

The gynecologic organs and the urinary tract system are intimately related in the pelvis. As a result, injuries to the urinary tract are inherent risks of gynecologic surgery. The bladder and the ureters are the most often injured or involved in the disease process. Technologic advances have significantly improved both the diagnostic and the therapeutic alternatives that are available for the management of vesical and ureteral injuries.

URETERIC INJURY

Epidemiology

Ureteral injuries can occur in several surgical settings but happen generally during retroperitoneal and pelvic surgeries. A meta-analysis concluded that hysterectomies are the cause of 54% of all surgical ureteric injuries.[1] Moreover, the incidence of ureteral lesions during a gynecologic procedure is reported to be between 0.5% and 1.5%.[1] The most common sites of injury are at the level of the uterine and ovarian arteries, the cardinal ligament, and the pelvic brim.[2] For the most part, an adequate knowledge of the anatomy will minimize the risk of ureteral trauma during pelvic surgery.

Risk factors

Several risk factors predispose to lesions of the ureter by a distortion of the anatomy, an involvement of the ureteral wall or a poor visibility during surgery. These risk factors are: the presence of malignancy or inflammatory process (endometriosis, pelvic inflammatory disease [PID]), the use of laparoscopic surgery, laser or electrocoagulation, a previous history of C-section or pelvic radiation therapy, and finally obesity and bleeding.

Presentation and evaluation

Several mechanisms may lead to ureteral injuries: ligature, laceration, crushing, stretching, and devascularization. A high level of suspicion during surgery is required to recognize a ureteral trauma. That is especially true for laparoscopic surgeries during which the tactile feeling of the structures is not as precise as it is for an open surgery. Moreover, the injury may not be identified as it may occur outside of the field of the camera. Aggressive intraoperative hydration, administration of diuretics and intravenous injection of 5 to 10 cc of indigo carmine dye will help to increase visualization of the ureters and therefore decrease the risk of trauma or at least contribute to identify the site of injury. Observation of the adventitia and of the peristalsis of the ureter are other means to evaluate the viability of the ureter after ureterolysis. In addition, preoperative ureteral stenting may help for the intraoperative recognition of ureteral injuries although it will not reduce the incidence of those injuries.[3,4] The risk of ureteral injuries at the time of stenting is one in 100 cases.[3] Failure of stent insertion on one side is known to be 13% and 2% for both sides.[3]

Ureteral traumas should be suspected during the postoperative period if the patient presents with flank pain, peritonitis, abdominal distension, de novo ascites, sepsis, prolonged ileus, hematuria, vaginal leakage secondary to ureterovaginal fistula, or rising serum creatinine levels. This increase of creatinine level results from an obstruction or reabsorption of intraperitoneal urine leakage. An intravenous pyelogram (IVP) can be performed, if a ureteral injury is suspected. However, the IVP findings are subtle and nonspecific: delayed renal function, ureteral deviation, ureteral dilatation, or ureteral nonvisualization. As much as 7% of IVPs are normal even in presence of a ureteral lesion.[2] Computed tomography (CT) can also be used in case where a ureteral injury is suspected. Delayed images are required to identify the possible extravasation of the contrast material. Other abdominal injuries may also be identified and it is possible to visualize hydronephrosis and quantified urinoma on CT scan images. False-negative results are relatively important and only a few published studies have assessed the accuracy of CT scans in a postoperative setting.[5] The utilization of magnetic resonance imaging has not been described to date. Retrograde and antegrade ureterographies may also be used to identify ureteral injuries. Those techniques will allow to assess both the level and the length of the lesion. Moreover, insertion of a ureteral stent may be simultaneously performed for treatment.

Treatment

The moment of recognition, the length of the defect, the anatomic location, the mechanism of injury, and the medical condition of the patient are the factors that will dictate the proper management of ureteral traumas. Intraoperative identification of ureteral injury requires immediate attention and there is no indication for surveillance management. Typically, these lesions are short in length, that is, less than 2 cm and subject to end-to-end repair (ureteroureterostomy) or ureteroneocystostomy. The suture on the ligated ureter should be removed and the ureter inspected for its viability. In doubt, the damaged segment of ureter should be resected and repaired over a ureteral stent with absorbable sutures. In most cases, partial or complete ureteral lacerations are better repaired using a complete anastomosis. Coagulation and laser injuries should also be carefully inspected. Heat diffusion may cause microthrombosis of adventitial vessels and frequently extends beyond macroscopically detectable margins, thus increasing the risk for ischemic injuries and late stenosis. Aperistaltic ureter with a well-preserved adventitia should be followed with imaging during the postoperative period to rule out hydronephrosis or stenosis. A devascularized ureter without laceration should be stented and followed over a long-term period after the removal of the stent.

Several basic principles should be applied during ureteral surgeries in order to increase the success rate. Careful mobilization of the injured ureter should be performed with a wide dissection to preserve the small ureteral vessels that are present in the adventitia. Debridement should be done until well-vascularized margins are reached. After spatulation of the ureter in order to increase the diameter of the anastomosis, a ureteral stent should be inserted and kept for 6 to 12 weeks (Figure 10-1). The repair should be tension-free, watertight and fine absorbable suture (5-0) should be used. Moreover, peritoneal or omental coverage of the anastomosis should be performed whenever possible. A Penrose or Jackson-Pratt drain should be placed in proximity to the repair and a urethral catheter inserted, if not already in place.

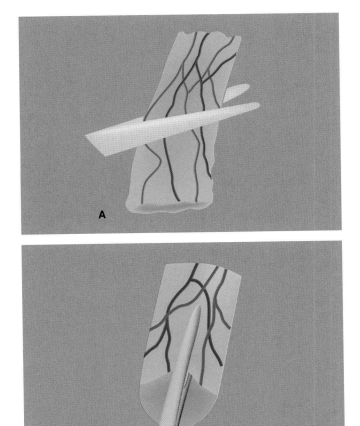

Figure 10-1 ■ Ureteroureterostomy.
A. Debridement of ureter. B. Spatulation of ureter. *(Continued)*

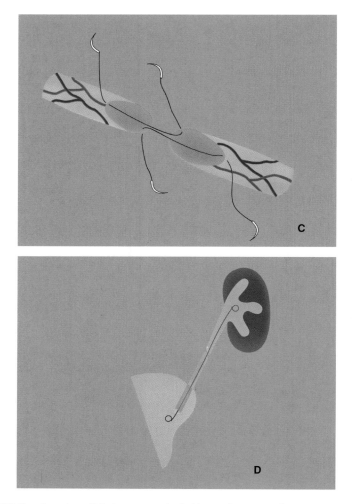

Figure 10-1 ■ *(continued)* C. Anastomosis. D. Ureteral stent in place.

Delayed ureteric injury recognition can be evaluated and treated with an endoscopic procedure. A retrograde pyelography and a stent insertion, with a separate drainage of the urinoma, may be attempted as a first line of treatment. Whenever unsuccessful, an antegrade approach via a percutaneous nephrostomy can be tried, although surgical management is generally the best option after failure of the endoscopic procedure. Open and laparoscopic approaches may also be planned. However, no published series have compared these two techniques. For an open procedure, the patient should be supine and a Pfannenstiel, Gibson, or midline incision may be performed. A flank position should be used, if the ureteral injury is repaired by laparoscopy. The use of three or four trocars is suggested. A careful mobilization of the ureter that may easily be found at the pelvis brim, resection of the injured part, debridement of the margins, spatulation of the ureter over 5 to 6 cm, stent insertion, tension-free, and watertight anastomosis with absorbable interrupted suture can all be performed during an open or laparoscopic surgery. Intra-abdominal suturing still remains the biggest challenge of the laparoscopic technique.

Tension-free anastomosis is not always possible to achieve during ureteroureterostomy which bridge up to 2 to 3 cm gaps after delicate mobilization and spatulation of the ureter. For cases where more length is required and for which the ureteral injury is adjacent to the bladder, an ureteroneocystostomy may be considered. No difference has been found between refluxing and nonrefluxing ureteral repairs in patients with a previous normal urinary tract.[6] Both intravesical (Politano-Leadbetter) and extravesical (Lich-Gregoir) ureteral reimplantations can be performed although the extravesical ureteroneocystostomy is simpler and avoids the need to widely open the bladder. Bladder mobilization in order to gain more length for injuries above the pelvic brim and to decrease tension on the anastomosis can be reached by performing a psoas hitch or a Boari flap. Other options for ureteral reconstruction include transureteroureterostomy, nephropexy, bowel interposition, renal autotransplantation, and nephrectomy. The indication and surgical techniques for those procedures are beyond the objective of this chapter.

For an antirefluxing extravesical reimplantation that is performed during a gynecologic procedure, the same ports may be used. One smooth grasper (Maryland), a needledriver, a pair of scissors, absorbable suture (Vicryl, Chromic, PDS, or Maxon), a ureteral stent with its guidewire, and an angiocatheter are the only instruments required for laparoscopic repair. Suturing devices such as the Endostich™ may also be employed. The detrusor muscle is incised longitudinally along the axis of the ureter in order to make a 3-cm tunnel for the ureter above the mucosa. The spatulated ureter is approximated to the bladder mucosa with interrupted sutures or two running sutures. The knots should be outside the bladder and a better visualization of the ureteral lumen is reached, if the needle comes from the inside of the lumen. The detrusor muscle fibers are then closed with three or four interrupted 3-0 sutures over the ureter to create the tunnel (Figure 10-2). The ureteral stent should be inserted on its guidewire through an angiocatheter after half the sutures are in place.

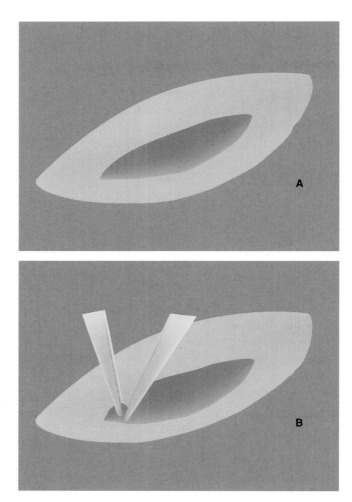

Figure 10-2 ▪ Extravesical reimplantation.
A. Incision of detrusor muscle. B. Opening of mucosa. *(Continued)*

Postoperative management

After a ureteral repair, large broad-spectrum antibiotic prophylaxis should be instituted. The urethral catheter may be safely removed 24 hours after the drain output subsides. Whenever there is an important drainage, the difference should be made between lymph and urine by measuring the creatinine level of the fluid. Antibiotics can be stopped after the urethral catheter and the drain are removed. The adequate position of the ureteral stent can be verified with a flat abdominal X-ray. The ureteral catheter may be removed by cystoscopy 6 to 12 weeks after the surgery.

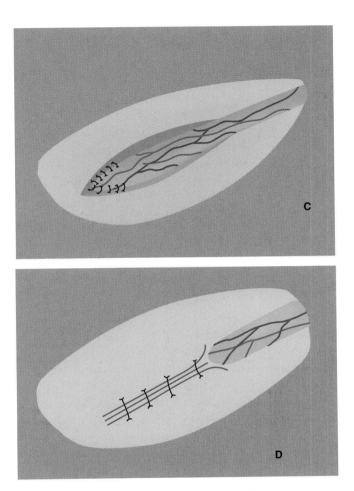

Figure 10-2 ■ *(continued)* C. Anastomosis of ureter. D. Closure of detrusor muscle to create ureteral tunnel.

Complications

Initial complications that are associated with ureteral repairs include infection, bleeding, and urine leakage. If urine leakage persists, the appropriate position of the ureteral stent should be confirmed and a urethral catheter should be kept on straight drainage, not only to decrease the ureteral reflux around the ureteral stent but also to maintain a low pressure in the urinary tract. Bladder spasms may lead to severe discomfort and are usually secondary to the presence of intravesical catheters. Anticholinergic medication may be prescribed in order to decrease the bladder contractions after a urinary tract infection is excluded. Ureterovaginal fistula may complicate gynecologic procedures or may present after ureteral surgeries. Endoscopic approaches have been described and are effective.[7] However, endoscopic management is not always possible. For that situation, laparoscopic ureteroneocystostomy is a safe, feasible, and effective option.[8] Late complications after a ureteral surgery are usually the result of ureteral stricture with hydronephrosis, lost of renal function or renal colic symptoms. Short ureteral stricture, less than 2 cm, may be managed by antegrade or retrograde endoscopic techniques including balloon dilatation or laserization under direct vision. Longer strictures will need an open surgical procedure to excise the scarred tissues and to reanastomose healthy ureteral margins.

BLADDER INJURY

Epidemiology

Among all organs of the urinary tract, the bladder is the most often injured during gynecological surgeries. The incidence of bladder trauma is evaluated between 0.3% and 1.6% and increases with the complexity of the surgery.[2] Since the advent of therapeutic laparoscopy, the incidence of iatrogenic bladder injuries has increased to 1.0 to 1.8 per 100 gynecologic cases.[2] The main differences between laparoscopic and open surgery which increase the risk of bladder perforation are the frequent use of laser or electrocoagulation and trocar insertion.

Risk factors

During gynecologic procedures, factors associated with increased risks of bladder injuries are similar to ureteral trauma, being the presence of malignancy, inflammatory process (endometriosis, PID), laparoscopic surgery, prior history of C-section, pelvic radiation therapy, use of laser, electrocoagulation, bladder distension, and bleeding.

Presentation and evaluation

Bladder injuries can be recognized intra- or postoperatively. At the time of surgery, vesical tears may be suspected or directly seen. Suspicion should be raised, if blood or carbon dioxide is seen in the urine bag during the procedure. Confirmation may be obtained by injection of diluted methylene blue via a urethral catheter followed by extravesical leakage. Bladder trauma should be suspected in the postoperative period if the patient presents with hematuria, inability to void, abdominal distension, de novo ascites, poor urine output with adequate intravascular volume, sepsis, prolonged ileus, or rising serum creatinine levels. Cystogram and CT-cystogram are the most adequate imaging modalities to diagnose vesical rupture. The use of 350 cc of dye is considered to be the appropriate volume to both detect significant leakage and to decrease the incidence of false-negative results. No relation has been found between the volume of leakage and the severity of the rupture. Vesical injuries are classified as extraperitoneal or intraperitoneal depending on the position of the laceration.

Treatment

The time of recognition, the anatomic position of the injury, and the medical condition of the patient dictate the proper management of bladder perforation. Conservative treatment may be offered to patients with delayed recognized extraperitoneal rupture without clot retention. Urethral catheterization with a large size catheter and antibiotic treatment with or without abdominal drainage are essential components of such treatment. Nonetheless, surgical primary closure of bladder injury decreases significantly the percentage of late complications.[9] The closure should be planned and performed as soon as recognized, intra- or postoperatively.

In a general trauma setting, bladder traumas are associated with 10% of ureteral traumas. This percentage is most likely lower for iatrogenic injuries but a high level of suspicion should be adopted as only one-third of ureteral lesions are identified during surgery. Intra- and postoperative evaluations of possible ureteral injuries have already been summarized previously in this chapter. Prior to primary repair, a careful evaluation of the anatomic position of the bladder injury should be performed. Lesions near the bladder neck and sphincter mechanisms as well as injuries close to the trigone, ureteral orifices or submucosal tunnel of the ureters should prompt urologic evaluation such as a cystoscopy, stent placement, or reconstructions other than simple closure.

Surgical treatment

Open and laparoscopic cystotomy repairs have been demonstrated to be equivalent for late results. When found intraoperatively, a laparoscopic iatrogenic bladder trauma can be safely repaired in a laparoscopic setting and then preserve the advantages of this technique.[10] Repair of simple bladder lacerations at the dome or on the anterior wall of the bladder can be performed by the gynecologist. However, repair of lesions of the base or of the posterior wall of the bladder should involve the urologist. As a matter of fact, these distal and posterior injuries can also affect the ureters and sphincter mechanisms, that need specialized evaluation and treatment. Additional trocars may be added to facilitate access to the laceration and to allow proper suturing of the defect but most of the time the ports that are already in place are sufficient to give adequate access for the repair. One simple smooth grasper, a needle holder, a pair of scissors, absorbable suture (Vicryl, Chromic, PDS, or Maxon), and the dexterity to perform intra-abdominal suturing are the only requirements to close cystotomy in laparoscopy. Alternatively, suturing devices such as the Endostich™ may be employed to facilitate endoscopic suturing without the need to position and grasp the needle. However, this device needs a 10-mm diameter port. The lateral trocars usually give the best access to the bladder for suturing. Traction on the bladder with an Alice or Babcock clamp to expose the injury may be performed through the suprapubic port.

Large spectrum antibiotics should be instituted and continued as long as both drain and catheter remain in place. A large size urethral catheter should be inserted, if not already in place, to permit drainage and intraoperative distension of the bladder. Bladder irrigation with normal saline with or without methylene blue, can be performed prior to closure to better identify the lesion. Absorbable suture (3-0 or 4-0) should be used for the repair, since permanent suture or staples can calcify intravesicaly, therefore leading to stone formation. Interrupted or running suture can be used and closure can be done in one (full thickness) or two lawyers (mucosa and muscularis) with similar results. Running sutures are usually preferred because fewer knots are needed and a better hemostasis is provided. Four basic principles should always be respected during bladder repair to help the healing process: unhealthy bladder margins should be debrided to reapproximate healthy mucosa, the closure should be tension-free, watertight and tissues like omentum or peritoneum should be secured on the repair to decrease the risk of fistulization. Synthetic glues may also be used to cover the repair and they have been evaluated safe for bladder mucosa.[11,12] After the closure is completed, bladder distension should be repeated to look for fluid leakage. A Penrose or a Jackson-Pratt drain should be positioned next to the bladder closure to clear any potential leakage and the urethral catheter must be checked regularly to insure proper drainage without clot retention. No significant advantages have been described for the additional use of a suprapubic catheter during the healing phase.[13]

Postoperative management

One week after the repair, 3-views voiding cystourethrography (VCUG) should be repeated to confirm proper healing of the bladder injury. If fluid leakage persists, the urethral catheter should be kept in place and the cystogram must be repeated a week later. The urethral catheter may be safely removed if the VCUG is normal. The abdominal drain can be pulled out 24 to 48 hours later, if no drainage occurs. The antibiotic prophylaxis may also be stopped at that point.

Complications

Despite a strict respect of repair principles, complications after bladder closure may occur. Fluid leakage is the most frequent complication that follows a cystotomy repair. Creatinine levels measurement can be performed on the fluid collected on the external drain. If the creatinine is higher than the serum level, the leakage is considered to be urine. If the creatinine level is similar to serum level, the leakage is most likely peritoneal or lymphatic fluid. Most of the times, urine leakage can be treated conservatively. One should make sure that the drainage of the urethral catheter is normal, without blood clots retention that would require a larger catheter and bladder irrigation. Adequate external drainage of urine leakage and the position of the drain should also be verified. Vesicovaginal fistula can also occur after a posterior wall bladder injury. Management can be conservative or surgical depending on the timing, severity and position of the fistula. Vesicovaginal fistula can be easily mistaken with urethral incontinence, another possible complication of bladder surgeries. Bladder hyperactivity may have an early or late presentation. An early onset of bladder spasms is not uncommon after a bladder surgery because of the presence of intravesical sutures and of a catheter. Urethral catheter drainage should be assessed to rule out blood clots retention and a urine culture should be performed. An evaluation of novel hyperactive symptoms after months of bladder repair, should allow to exclude bladder stones that may grow on nonabsorbable sutures. Finally, ureteral obstruction can complicate vesical surgery. Edema, ligature, or kinking of the ureter may cause renal colic pain with new hydronephrosis. Antegrade or retrograde endoscopic management with a ureteral stent is the first line of treatment, although open surgery may be mandatory, if endoscopic techniques fail.

CONCLUSION

Iatrogenic surgical traumas or involvement of the urinary tract system during treatment of gynecologic diseases are fairly common. Prevention will always be the best scenario and appropriate knowledge of the pelvic anatomy and of the risk factors for urinary injuries are the best tools for the surgeon. Technical advancements in laparoscopic surgery now permit to repair the urinary tract lesions with similar success rates than for open surgeries while preserving the advantages of laparoscopy.

REFERENCES

1. St Lezin MA, Stoller ML. Surgical ureteral injuries. *Urology*. 1991;38(6):497–506.
2. Mammen C, Chilaka V, Cust MP. Urological surgical techniques. *Best Pract Res Clin Obstet Gynaecol*. 2006;20(1):139-156.
3. Bothwell WN, Bleicher RJ, Dent TL. Prophylactic ureteral catheterization in colon surgery. A five-year review. *Dis Colon Rectum*. 1994;37(4):330–334.
4. Kuno K, Menzin A, Kauder HH, Sison C, Gal D. Prophylactic ureteral catheterization in gynecologic surgery. *Urology*. 1998;52(6):1004–1008.
5. Gayer G, Hertz M, Zissin R. Ureteral injuries: CT diagnosis. *Semin Ultrasound CT MR*. 2004;25(3):277–285.
6. Stefanovic KB, Bukurov NS, Marinkovic JM. Non-antireflux versus antireflux ureteroneocystostomy in adults. *Br J Urol*. 1991;67(3):263–266.
7. Narang V, Sinha T, Karan SC, et al. Ureteroscopy: Savior to the gynecologist? Ureteroscopic management of post laparoscopic-assisted vaginal hysterectomy ureterovaginal fistulas. *J Minim Invasive Gynecol*. 2007;14(3):345–347.
8. Modi P, Goel R, Dodiya S. Laparoscopic ureteroneocystostomy for distal ureteral injuries. *Urology*. 2005;66(4):751–753.
9. Kotkin L, Koch MO. Morbidity associated with nonoperative management of extraperitoneal bladder injuries. *J Trauma*. 1995;38(6):895–898.
10. Nezhat CH, Seidman DS, Nezhat F, Rottenberg H, Nezhat C. Laparoscopic management of intentional and unintentional cystotomy. *J Urol*. 1996;156(4):1400–1402.
11. Seifman BD, Rubin MA, Williams AL, Wolf JS. Use of absorbable cyanoacrylate glue to repair an open cystotomy. *J Urol*. 2002;167(4):1872–1875.
12. Evans LA, Ferguson KH, Foley JP, Rozanski TA, Morey AF. Fibrin sealant for the management of genitourinary injuries, fistulas and surgical complications. *J Urol*. 2003;169(4):1360–1362.
13. Alli MO, Singh B, Moodley J, Shaik AS. Prospective evaluation of combined suprapubic and urethral catheterization to urethral drainage alone for intraperitoneal bladder injuries. *J Trauma*. 2003;55(6):1152–1154.

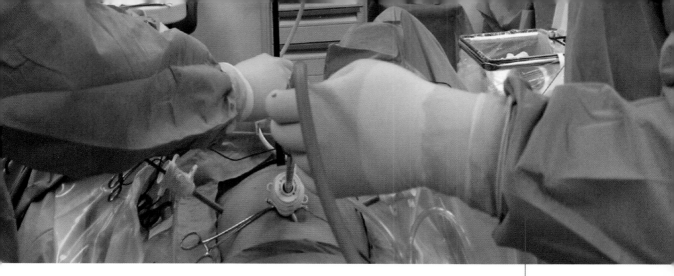

MISCELLANEOUS, INCLUDING OMENTECTOMY, APPENDECTOMY, LYSIS ADHESIONS, AND SPLENECTOMY

11

Jan Hauspy, Rachel Kupets, and Allan L. Covens

Indications/contraindications will be discussed for each procedure separately in this chapter. *Setup, patient positioning, and equipment* procedures described in this chapter can be part of a gynecologic oncologic operation. Since omentectomy, appendectomy, lysis of adhesions, and splenectomy are rarely the primary goal of the operation for a gynecologic oncologist, the setup, positioning, and use of equipment will be dictated by the intent of the primary operation. Ideally, for the abovementioned procedures, we prefer to position the patient in dorsolithotomy with both legs in stirrups. A Foley catheter is inserted in the bladder at the start of the operation. Trocar port locations: one midline 10- to 12-mm trocar supra- or infraumbilically, a second midline 10- to 12-mm trocar suprapubically, and two 5-mm ports 2-cm medial and cranial of the left and right anterior superior iliac spines. *Pre- and postoperative management and complications* will be discussed according to the individual procedures.

OMENTECTOMY

Indications/contraindications

In patients with gynecologic malignancies, omentectomy is very often performed as part of a staging procedure. Omentectomy will be performed for staging or debulking of ovarian, primary peritoneal, and fallopian tube cancers. The use of laparoscopy for staging and/or debulking of these tumors is controversial. Since debulking procedures for ovarian/primary peritoneal/fallopian tube cancers are not routinely performed laparoscopically, a more common scenario is the removal of omentum as part of a staging procedure for endometrial cancer. Mobilization of the omentum is sometimes performed for procedures, in which the serosa of the rectosigmoid colon is repaired or as a protective patch after complicated pelvic surgery.

Setup, patient positioning, and equipment

Omentectomy is rarely the primary goal of a gynecologic operation; hence, the placement of the trocar ports if often decided by the intent of the primary operation. Ideally, for laparoscopic omentectomy we prefer to position the patient in dorsolithotomy with both legs in stirrups. Port locations are as follows: in the midline a 10- or 12-mm trocar supra- or infraumbilically, a second midline 10- or 12-mm trocar suprapubically and two 5-mm ports in the mid-clavicular line, at the level of the umbilicus. Alternatively, for the lateral 5-mm ports, insertions can be made approximately 2 cm medial and cranial of the anterior superior iliac spine. The latter approach, however, may compromise reach of the instruments in the upper abdomen (especially at the greater curvature of the stomach) and because these lower lateral ports can limit your mobility to work in the upper abdomen because of interference of the patient's legs. At least one monitor should be placed at the cranial end of the patient. The camera-scope is inserted in the lower/suprapubic trocar port, with the operating table leveled or in slight reversed Trendelenburg position.

Infracolic omentectomy or omental biopsies are relatively easy to perform when no adhesions are present. A grasper is used through the umbilical port to elevate the omentum. Depending on the placement and size of the omentum, a grasper will be placed in one of the lateral ports, holding the omentum under traction between the two instruments. The greater omentum is detached from the transverse colon, up to the splenic flexure. Gentle traction on the transverse colon can be applied with an atraumatic grasper. Ultrasonic dissectors or electrothermal bipolar vessel sealers provide an easy and safe way to divide the omentum. Traction-countertraction is essential for a smooth laparoscopic division of the omentum. Monopolar electrocautery devices should be avoided because of a higher risk of conduction and thermal damage to the transverse colon. The current flow of monopolar cautery is unpredictable and can result in thermal damage distant from the point of contact.

By detaching the omentum from the transverse colon, the lesser sac is exposed. In order to perform a supracolic omentectomy, the blood supply to the omentum branching of the left and right gastroepiploic arteries have to be identified and coagulated/sealed along the greater curvature of the stomach. Alternatively, a vascular endoscopic stapler can be used to staple across the base of the omentum along the greater curvature of the stomach. Multiple loads have to be used and therefore, this approach can be more time consuming. A 10- to 12-mm port is needed for the latter approach. Detachment of the omentum at the level of the splenic flexure can be tedious. Traction should be applied with caution, as too much traction can potentially result in splenic injury with significant bleeding. Increasing reversed Trendelenburg position combined with a right lateral tilt, can improve visualization of the omentum at the spleen.

In a patient with prior surgical procedures, the omentum is often adherent to the anterior abdominal wall. When good visualization of the surrounding structures is obtained, we often use these adhesions to our advantage as the omentum is automatically suspended, making the traction-countertraction easier.

Pre- and postoperative management

For optimal visualization of the omentum and stomach, a nasogastric tube can be inserted by the anesthesiologist at the start of the procedure.

No specific postoperative management is necessary for patients who underwent an omentectomy as part of their operation. Unless otherwise indicated, the nasogastric tube can be removed at the end of the procedure.

Complications

The most common complications of omentectomy are bleeding and bowel injury. While mobilizing the omentum, injury to the spleen can occur. The ultrasonic dissector (harmonic scalpel) or electrothermal bipolar vessel sealer devices (Ligasure device) reduce conduction, thereby minimizing the risk of bowel trauma.[1] Thermal trauma is more commonly seen with the use of monopolar electrocautery.[2,3] Bowel trauma by conduction is often missed at laparoscopy and has a delayed and covert presentation.[4] The consequences of unrecognized bowel trauma can be detrimental[5] and often require reoperation with possible bowel resection and/or colostomy.[2] It is, therefore, imperative to take great precaution while using electrocautery in the abdomen. At the end of the omentectomy careful inspection of the omental edge and transverse colon should be performed.

| APPENDECTOMY

Indications

Women with primary appendiceal cancer often present with ovarian metastases and initial surgery will often be performed by a gynecologic oncologist because of presumed ovarian pathology.[6] The appendix should always be examined on any routine laparoscopy but certainly in the presence of ovarian masses. Appendectomy is not recommended routinely for staging of early stage (apparent stages I and II) serous ovarian cancer,[7,8] but the appendix can sometimes be involved with metastatic tumor in advanced ovarian cancer and as such has to be removed as part of the cytoreductive surgery. When mucinous tumors of the ovary are diagnosed intraoperatively, even a normal looking appendix should be removed. If primary appendiceal cancer is confirmed, a right hemicolectomy should be performed, rather than a simple appendectomy.

For abnormal appearing appendices or in patients with coinciding appendicitis, appendectomy is warranted.

Contraindications

Even though the added morbidity of appendectomy to any larger operation is limited, routine removal of the appendix during gynecologic cancer staging is not recommended.[7,8]

Setup, patient positioning, and equipment

In gynecologic oncology, appendectomy is often performed as part of a more extensive operation, such as removal of a pelvic mass or hysterectomy, hence the placement of the trocar ports will often be tailored toward the intent of the primary operation. Ideally, for laparoscopic appendectomy the camera is inserted through an umbilical port and a 10- or 12-mm suprapubic port is in place with one or two lateral 5-mm trocar ports.

In the case of appendicitis, the omentum will often be adherent to the appendix and may need to be removed for visualization of the appendix. Careful inspection of the area is warranted to assess the degree of inflammation surrounding the appendix. Retrocecal appendices may not be visualized by just manipulating the cecum and require mobilization of the cecum and ascending colon for proper exposure. The appendix can then be traced by opening the retroperitoneal space over the psoas muscle, lateral to the ascending colon. Localization of the right ureter and infunibulopelvic vessels should be performed in order to safely mobilize the cecum and ascending colon. The location of the tip of the appendix can vary significantly. When the tip is not easily found, the appendiceal base can more consistently be identified (2–3 cm inferolateral to the ileocecal junction). After identifying the appendix, the tip will be gently grasped with an atraumatic grasper and elevated towards the anterior abdominal wall. This allows for removal of any adherent omentum and gentle removal of adhesions.

Gentle medial traction with an atraumatic grasper can be applied to the cecum for better exposure. After isolation of the appendix and removal of any adherent tissue, the mesoappendix is divided at the base of the appendix. Several techniques can be applied. If available, an ultrasonic dissector (harmonic scalpel) or electrothermal bipolar vessel sealer devices (Ligasure device) can ligate and divide the mesoappendix, including the appendicular artery. Alternatively, with endoscissors, a small opening can be created in the mesoappendix at the base of the appendix. The mesoappendix and appendicular artery can than be clipped with hemoclips or coagulated with bipolar diathermy and divided with endoscissors. Gentle removal of the fat around the base of the appendix is than performed to create a free space at the base of the appendix, sufficient to tie off the appendix. The base of the appendix is tied of with an endoloop pretied suture at the base and a second loop 1 cm distally. With scissors, the appendix is cut in between the sutures, leaving slightly more residual at the proximal end.

In the general setup for gynecologic laparoscopic procedures, often a 12-mm suprapubic trocar port is present, allowing for the introduction of a linear endoscopic stapler. With this technique, a vascular endoscopic stapler is applied and fired across the base of the appendix including the mesoappendix. When the mesoappendix is too bulky, a two-step procedure can be used, creating a window at the base of the appendix, as described above and using a vascular stapler for the mesoappendix and an intestinal stapler across the appendix proper. In the absence of a 12-mm suprapubic port, this technique can still be performed using the umbilical port to insert the stapler and one of the 5-mm ports with a 5-mm camera scope. Stapling the appendix is safe and quick and allows for minimal manipulation of the appendix, reducing the risk for bleeding and rupture. This technique can also safely be applied in the case of an incarcerated appendix or when the base of the appendix is necrotic or inflamed. The stapler can then be partially applied across the base of the cecum in healthy tissue rather than cutting across the necrotic base, thereby reducing the risk of postoperative rupture. When the tip of the appendix is buried, it is often safer to divide the base of the appendix before attempting to remove the adhesions around the tip. This allows for gentle traction of the base of the appendix without risk of rupturing the base or disrupting the appendicular blood supply.

With an average-sized appendix, the specimen can often be removed through the 12-mm trocar port. The appendix is firmly grasped at the proximal end of the specimen and can usually be pulled safely through the 12-mm port. In the event of an enlarged or bulky appendix, an endoscopic bag can be used to remove the specimen. When appendectomy is part of a total hysterectomy, the appendix can be removed through the vagina after the uterus has been removed.

Complications

Abscess formation is a well recognized complication from laparoscopic appendectomy and can usually be managed by percutaneous drainage and antibiotics.[9,10] Abscesses are usually formed after appendectomy for appendicitis and may be seen more with aggressive manipulation of the inflamed appendix.[10] Injury to the ascending colon and terminal ileum can occur during manipulation of the appendix. Complications are more often seen in the presence of appendicitis or an incarcerated appendix.

ADHESIOLYSIS

Indications

Mechanical injury and ischemia of the peritoneum during surgical procedures can result in formation of abnormal fibrous structures in the abdomen known as adhesions. Peritoneal adhesions are found most commonly in patients with prior surgeries[11] or with a history of pelvic/abdominal inflammatory diseases. In a Scottish epidemiologic study, readmission for adhesions within 1 year after gynecologic surgery was approximately 1%, with similar readmission rates after laparoscopy and laparotomy. Peritoneal adhesions can be the cause of infertility, abdominal pain, and intestinal obstructions.[12] The majority of small bowel obstructions are caused by postoperative adhesion formation,[13,14] mostly seen after colorectal surgery.

Adhesiolysis is most often performed for treatment of infertility or in patients with chronic pelvic pain. There is evidence to suggest an improved pregnancy rate in the former, however, no clear advantage has been shown for treatment of chronic pelvic pain. A number of patients who undergo surgery for gynecologic cancers will have adhesions, not always in the presence of clinical symptoms. Patients with midline incisions tend to have more adhesions than patients who underwent a Pfannenstiel incision and patients who have undergone surgery for gynecologic reasons tend to have more adhesions than when the surgery was performed for obstetric reasons.[15] Laparoscopy significantly reduces the chance of postoperative adhesions if compared to laparotomy.[16,17] A study by the Operative Laparoscopy Study Group assessed adhesion reformation and "de novo" adhesion formation after laparoscopic adhesiolysis. "De novo" formation after laparoscopy is relatively uncommon (~10%), however, adhesion reformation after laparoscopic adhesiolysis occurs in the majority of patients (~97%). The main goal of adhesiolysis in gynecologic oncology patients is improved access, and visualization of the operation field.

Contraindications

A relative contraindication for starting a laparoscopic procedure is the presence of extensive adhesions as seen in patients after extensive bowel surgery and/or postoperative intraperitoneal infections.

Setup, patient positioning, and equipment

Expected extensive intra-abdominal adhesions may be a relative contraindication for performing laparoscopy. However, it is often very difficult if not impossible to accurately assess the extent of adhesions preoperatively. Adhesiolysis in gynecologic oncology is seldom the primary goal of the operation. Therefore, the port placement is often dictated by the intended surgery. Even though the optimal location for insertion of a Verres needle is around the umbilicus because of the proximity of the skin to the fascial layer, in patients with prior incisions in the vicinity of the umbilicus or in patients with umbilical hernias, alternative Verres needle insertion in the left upper quadrant or open access trocar placement may be safer.[18] The left upper quadrant insertion is performed on the midclavicular line, just below the rib cage. This area rarely exhibits adhesions and the peritoneum is attached to the ribs, reducing peritoneal tenting on insertion. Prior to entry at this level, a nasogastric tube should be inserted to deflate the stomach and decrease the risk of accidental gastric injury. This is important, particularly in patients who had a difficult intubation with possible insufflation of air in the stomach. A needle laparoscope can be inserted prior to inserting a larger trocar.

Equipment for the dissection of adhesions varies. In most cases, simple dissection with endoscopic scissors in areas of filmy, loose adhesions is preferable. Monopolar coagulation usually suffices to control bleeding, however, the risk of lateral electrical spread with limited visualization or distant injuries because of insulation defects is higher than bipolar techniques. No trials have been performed to assess the different effects of monopolar, bipolar, ultrascission or vessel sealing devices on reformation of adhesions. One of the advantages of vessel sealing devices in adhesiolysis, is that one instrument can function as a coagulation device as well as a pair of scissors with both components usable separately. With this ergonomical advantage and the limited lateral spread of the electrical current, vessel sealing devices can safely reduce time spent on adhesiolysis. Atraumatic graspers are useful to manipulate bowel during adhesiolysis.

Pre- and postoperative management

The value of adjuvants to prevent formation of peritoneal adhesions is controversial, despite their widespread use. Corticosteriods, antibiotics, nonsteroidal anti-inflammatory drugs, Dextran 70, and surgical membranes have all been suggested to improve postoperative formation of adhesions. Most of the above-mentioned products, have questionable efficacy and some products may have potential adverse effects such as delayed wound healing with corticosteroids and allergic reactions to other agents. A Cochrane database review concluded that barrier agents seem to reduce de novo formation and reformation of adhesions, but there is no evidence of any impact on pelvic pain, and insufficient data to support its use to improve pregnancy rates.[19]

Complications

Because of adhesions, injuries at the start of the operation while creating the pneumoperitoneum and during trocar placement are more common. Secondly, organ injury caused by taking down adhesion can be seen as a result of traction and/or thermal damage. When unexpected adhesions are found on entry of the abdomen, careful inspection of the abdomen is warranted to identify possible entry injuries.

SPLENECTOMY

Indications

The most common scenario in gynecologic oncology that requires splenectomy would be in a patient with ovarian cancer, in the presence of omental caking extending to the spleen. This scenario usually appears in patients with bulky disease and warrants extensive exploration of the abdomen for other disease sites including palpation of the diaphragms, pelvic, and para-aortic lymph node basins, kidneys, liver surface, etc. In the majority of these patients, laparoscopy is contraindicated. In rare occasions a focal isolated implant/recurrence of ovarian cancer on the spleen may require splenectomy[20] or when the spleen is injured during initial surgery as a result of an omentectomy.

Contraindications

Severe coagulopathy or thrombocytopenia, severe splenomegaly, and a calcified splenic artery are contraindications for performing splenectomy laparoscopically.

Setup, patient positioning, and equipment

The technique of laparoscopic splenectomy has evolved over the last years. Initial reports described this procedure in supine position,[21,22] however, more recently a lateral approach has become more used with the patient in right decubitus or "leaning" position.[23–25] Even with the anterior approach, the procedure will involve right lateral tilt and reverse-Trendelenburg of the operating table to allow gravity to move other organs away from the left upper quadrant, simultaneously suspending the spleen for optimal access. A 30-degree or 45-degree scope is needed for optimal visualization. One or two monitors are placed at the head-side of the operating table. Port placement varies and can be adjusted to fit the rest of the procedure, if splenectomy is not the sole purpose of the operation. Ideally, four to five ports are used. A 10- to 12-mm supraumbilical port, a 5-mm subxiphoid port and a 5-mm right lateral port (in between the umbilical and subxiphoid ports), usually placed slightly more superior than for a typical gynecologic setup. The latter port can function simultaneously for the splenectomy and for access to the pelvis. Two left lateral ports, one in the mid-clavicular line and one more laterally are placed as the surgeons' working ports. One port should be able to accommodate a stapling device (10–12 mm port).

A large endoscopy bag to fit the whole spleen is used.

Pre- and postoperative management

When splenectomy is electively planned as a single operation or part of another procedure, preoperative measures include assessment of availability of blood products and vaccination against overwhelming post-splenectomy infection. The pneumococcal vaccine should be administered (preferably prior to surgery) to all patients who are planned for splenectomy. Nasogastric tube insertion is only recommended when great difficulty is encountered during dissection of the short gastric vessels.

Complications

Bleeding can occur during laparoscopic splenectomy and can be hard to control, sometimes necessitating conversion to laparotomy.[26] Splenosis is rare but can present several years after splenic surgery as an intra-abdominal mass or port site splenosis.[27–30] Even though laparoscopic splenectomy is feasible in patients with giant spleens, the complication rates seem to be correlated to size.[31]

▎RESULTS—SMALL REVIEW OF THE LITERATURE

The transverse colon is retracted caudally and the greater curvature of the stomach is retracted cranio-medially. First, the inferior pole of the spleen is cleared. The splenico-colic ligament, pancreatico-splenic ligament, and lieno-renal ligaments are divided. The use of an ultrasonic dissector (harmonic scalpel) or electrothermal bipolar vessel sealer devices (Ligasure device) facilitates ligation of these ligaments. Alternatively, a linear vascular stapler can be used to perform these dissections. In a small number of patients, arteries originating in the left gastro epiploic can be found at the inferior splenic pole. The next step of the splenectomy is the division of the splenic vessels at the hilum. Because of the size of the splenic vessels, a vascular stapler is necessary as these vessels are usually over the size limit that is considered safe of ultranonic or vessel sealer devices. The only remaining medial attachments are the gastrosplenic ligaments, containing the short gastric vessels. These can be dissected with ultrasonic or vessel sealer devices. At this stage, the spleen should be completely detached. Great caution should be exercised not to fragment the spleen during the procedure. Similarly, for extraction of the spleen careful manipulation of the spleen is necessary. The spleen is placed into a large endobag and can be removed in pieces with a grasper pulling fragments of the spleen through the 12-mm port.

REFERENCES

1. Entezari K, Hoffmann P, Goris M, Peltier A, Van Velthoven R. A review of currently available vessel sealing systems. *Minim Invasive Ther Allied Technol.* 2007;16(1):52-57.
2. Chapron C, Pierre F, Harchaoui Y, Lacroix S, Beguin S, Querleu D, et al. Gastrointestinal injuries during gynaecological laparoscopy. *Hum Reprod.* 1999;14(2): 333-337.
3. Tulikangas PK, Smith T, Falcone T, Boparai N, Walters MD. Gross and histologic characteristics of laparoscopic injuries with four different energy sources. *Fertil Steril.* 2001;75(4):806-810.
4. Vilos GA. Laparoscopic bowel injuries: Forty litigated gynaecological cases in Canada. *J Obstet Gynaecol Can.* 2002;24(3):224-230.
5. Lo KW, Yuen P. Mortality following laparoscopic surgery. *Gynecol Obstet Invest.* 1999;48(3):203-204.
6. Dietrich CS III, Desimone CP, Modesitt SC, Depriest PD, Ueland FR, Pavlik EJ, et al. Primary appendiceal cancer: Gynecologic manifestations and treatment options. *Gynecol Oncol.* 2007;104(3):602-606.
7. Ramirez PT, Slomovitz BM, McQuinn L, Levenback C, Coleman RL. Role of appendectomy at the time of primary surgery in patients with early-stage ovarian cancer. *Gynecol Oncol.* 2006;103(3):888-890.
8. Bese T, Kosebay D, Kaleli S, Oz AU, Demirkiran F, Gezer A. Appendectomy in the surgical staging of ovarian carcinoma. *Int J Gynaecol Obstet.* 1996;53(3):249-252.

9. Tang E, Ortega AE, Anthone GJ, Beart RW Jr. Intra-abdominal abscesses following laparoscopic and open appendectomies. *Surg Endosc* 1996;10(3):327–328.

10. Gupta R, Sample C, Bamehriz F, Birch DW. Infectious complications following laparoscopic appendectomy. *Can J Surg*. 2006;49(6):397–400.

11. Lehmann-Willenbrock E, Mecke H, Riedel HH. Sequelae of appendectomy, with special reference to intra-abdominal adhesions, chronic abdominal pain, and infertility. *Gynecol Obstet Invest*. 1990;29(4):241–245.

12. Vrijland WW, Jeekel J, van Geldorp HJ, Swank DJ, Bonjer HJ. Abdominal adhesions: Intestinal obstruction, pain, and infertility. *Surg Endosc*. 2003;17(7):1017–1022.

13. Al-Took S, Platt R, Tulandi T. Adhesion-related small-bowel obstruction after gynecologic operations. *Am J Obstet Gynecol*. 1999;180(2 Pt 1):313–315.

14. Nieuwenhuijzen M, Reijnen MM, Kuijpers JH, van Goor H. Small bowel obstruction after total or subtotal colectomy: A 10-year retrospective review. *Br J Surg*. 1998;85(9):1242–1245.

15. Brill AI, Nezhat F, Nezhat CH, Nezhat C. The incidence of adhesions after prior laparotomy: A laparoscopic appraisal. *Obstet Gynecol*. 1995;85(2):269–272.

16. Lundorff P, Hahlin M, Kallfelt B, Thorburn J, Lindblom B. Adhesion formation after laparoscopic surgery in tubal pregnancy: A randomized trial versus laparotomy. *Fertil Steril*. 1991;55(5):911–915.

17. Garrard CL, Clements RH, Nanney L, Davidson JM, Richards WO. Adhesion formation is reduced after laparoscopic surgery. *Surg Endosc*. 1999;13(1):10–13.

18. Vilos GA, Ternamian A, Dempster J, Laberge PY. Laparoscopic entry: A review of techniques, technologies, and complications. *J Obstet Gynaecol Can*. 2007; 29(5):433–447.

19. Farquhar C, Vandekerckhove P, Watson A, Vail A, Wiserman D. Barrier agents for preventing adhesions after surgery for subfertility. *Cochrane Database Syst Rev*. 1999(1).

20. Otrock ZK, Seoud MA, Khalifeh MJ, Makarem JA, Shamseddine AI. Laparoscopic splenectomy for isolated parenchymal splenic metastasis of ovarian cancer. *Int J Gynecol Cancer*. 2006;16(5):1933–1935.

21. Silecchia G, Boru CE, Fantini A, Raparelli L, Greco F, Rizzello M, et al. Laparoscopic splenectomy in the management of benign and malignant hematologic diseases. *JSLS*. 2006;10(2):199–205.

22. Park A, Targarona EM, Trias M. Laparoscopic surgery of the spleen: State of the art. *Langenbecks Arch Surg*. 2001;386(3):230–239.

23. Palanivelu C, Jani K, Malladi V, Shetty R, Senthilkumar R, Maheshkumar G. Early ligation of the splenic artery in the leaning spleen approach to laparoscopic splenectomy. *J Laparoendosc Adv Surg Tech A*. 2006;16(4):339–344.

24. Tan M, Zheng CX, Wu ZM, Chen GT, Chen LH, Zhao ZX. Laparoscopic splenectomy: The latest technical evaluation. *World J Gastroenterol*. 2003;9(5):1086–1089.

25. Hashizume M, Tanoue K, Akahoshi T, Morita M, Ohta M, Tomikawa M, et al. Laparoscopic splenectomy: The latest modern technique. *Hepatogastroenterology*. 1999;46(26):820–824.

26. Katkhouda N, Hurwitz MB, Rivera RT, Chandra M, Waldrep DJ, Gugenheim J, et al. Laparoscopic splenectomy: Outcome and efficacy in 103 consecutive patients. *Ann Surg.* 1998;228(4):568–578.

27. Kumar RJ, Borzi PA. Splenosis in a port site after laparoscopic splenectomy. *Surg Endosc.* 2001;15(4):413–414.

28. Khosravi MR, Margulies DR, Alsabeh R, Nissen N, Phillips EH, Morgenstern L. Consider the diagnosis of splenosis for soft tissue masses long after any splenic injury. *Am Surg.* 2004;70(11):967–970.

29. Sikov WM, Schiffman FJ, Weaver M, Dyckman J, Shulman R, Torgan P. Splenosis presenting as occult gastrointestinal bleeding. *Am J Hematol.* 2000;65(1):56–61.

30. Dwyer NT, Whelan TF. Renal splenosis presenting as a renal mass. *Can J Urol.* 2005;12(3):2710–2712.

31. Patel AG, Parker JE, Wallwork B, Kau KB, Donaldson N, Rhodes MR, et al. Massive splenomegaly is associated with significant morbidity after laparoscopic splenectomy. *Ann Surg.* 2003;238(2):235–240.

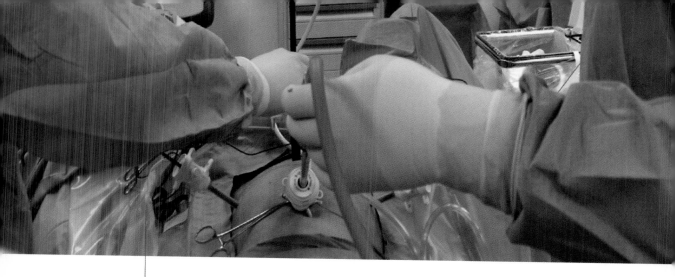

12 ANESTHESIA FOR LAPAROSCOPIC GYNECOLOGICAL SURGERY

Alayne Kealey

Gynecologists have been performing laparoscopic surgery routinely since the 1970s. Over the years, the improvements to instruments and innovative techniques have allowed minimal access surgery to evolve even further. In addition to gynecological procedures, laparoscopic colorectal, hepatobiliary, gastroesophageal, and urologic surgeries, are now common.

Laparoscopic techniques have gained popularity in part because of the reports of a reduction in postoperative pain, less postoperative pulmonary complications and better postoperative respiratory function, less postoperative wound infection, a reduction in length of hospital stay, and faster return to work.[1] Although minimal access surgery is often referred to as *minimally invasive*, the term can be misleading. The creation of a pneumoperitoneum to facilitate surgical technique can compromise the cardiorespiratory function of patients, and consequently, serious morbidity and fatalities have occurred during laparoscopic surgery.[2] The increasing age and comorbidities seen in the patients that are presenting for minimal access surgeries make providing anesthesia for this population more challenging, as does the increasing number of outpatient procedures. However, the benefits of laparoscopic surgery often outweigh the potential complications.

In this chapter, the anesthetic considerations for laparoscopic gynecological surgery will be reviewed. To begin, preoperative considerations and contraindications to minimal access surgery will be discussed. Next, the intraoperative anesthetic management of these patients will be examined, including the physiologic changes associated with the pneumoperitoneum and patient position, as well as the potential complications from laparoscopic surgery and their management. Finally, the chapter will conclude with a look at analgesic options and other postoperative issues.

PREOPERATIVE CONSIDERATIONS

The patient population presenting for laparoscopic gynecological surgery is relatively heterogeneous, ranging from healthy young women for an oophrectomy to older adults or very sick patients for complex laparoscopic hysterectomies and cancer staging. Preoperative anesthetic evaluation provides valuable information on perioperative risk, and can anticipate the need for specialized anesthesia techniques or a monitored bed in the postoperative period. Meeting the anesthesiologist can also diminish the anxiety that patients feel regarding the upcoming surgery and general anesthetic,[3] and they can be counseled about analgesia and ambulatory surgery.

The purpose of the preoperative anesthetic evaluation is to identify and reduce the risks associated with anesthesia and surgery. The American Society of Anesthesiology (ASA) classification system, upon which the current preoperative evaluation is based, is a modification of a first attempt to quantify risks associated with surgery, undertaken in 1941.[4] The system estimated anesthesia-related mortality, but was based solely on associated preoperative medical condition, without consideration for type of anesthesia or nature of surgery. Initially, four categories were established—ASA 1, with the lowest risk of mortality, to ASA 4, with the highest expected mortality. A more recent modification adds the ASA 5 category, for patients who are expected to die shortly with or without surgery. Studies have demonstrated a correlation between ASA status and perioperative mortality, but that ASA status does not necessarily help predict other complications[4] nor does it take surgical risk into account. On the other hand, the American Heart Association and American College of Cardiology (AHA/ACC) guidelines for preoperative assessment of the cardiac patient for noncardiac surgery allows for risk evaluation and suggest preoperative evaluation based on both patient medical comorbidities and surgical risk.[5] As the delay of some procedures may compromise the oncologic care of the patient, proceeding with surgery also depends on whether the delay will allow for a perioperative risk reduction or simply postpone the inevitable.

Healthy individuals for low-risk surgical procedures generally do not require a preanesthesia consultation—an evaluation in the holding area on the day of surgery is usually sufficient. However, based on the planned surgery or comorbid disease, certain patients do require assessment prior to the day of their surgery (Table 12-1).

Contraindications to laparoscopic surgery

Those patients who are at highest risk of perioperative complications, often benefit the most from minimal access surgery. They include patients with cardiac or respiratory compromise, morbid obesity, and the older adults. Special care, however, must be taken with anesthesia and surgical technique.

Regardless of perioperative care, absolute contraindications to laparoscopic surgery exist (Table 12-2). They include shock, markedly increased intracranial pressure (ICP), severe myopia or retinal detachment, and inadequate surgical equipment or monitoring devices.[6] Patients with an increased ICP from a closed head injury or space-occupying lesion have been shown to have abrupt intracranial hypertension within minutes of pneumoperitoneum, because of the increased intrathoracic pressure and impaired venous drainage of the lumbar venous pressure.[7]

Relative contraindications to laparoscopic surgery include bullous emphysema, a history of spontaneous pneumothorax, pregnancy, life-threatening emergencies, prolonged laparoscopy more than of 6 hours (associated with acidosis), and new laparoscopic procedures.[6] Laparoscopic surgery can be safely performed in patients with ventriculo-peritoneal (VP) shunts, but shunt function should be checked, with visualization of free CSF drainage from distal end of the catheter, and the lowest pressure and shortest necessary period of abdominal insufflation should be used.[8] For laparoscopic surgery in the pregnant patient, complications can be minimized by delaying surgery until the second trimester, considering an open technique and alternate sites for entry into the peritoneum, and keeping the patient in a level position with left lateral tilt.[9]

Table 12-1	**CONDITIONS FOR WHICH PREOPERATIVE EVALUATION MAY BE RECOMMENDED BEFORE THE DAY OF SURGERY**[*]

General
  Medical condition inhibiting ability to engage in normal daily activity.
  Medical condition necessitating continual assistance or monitoring at home within the past 6 months.
  Admission within the past 2 months for acute or exacerbation of chronic condition.
Cardiocirculatory
  History of angina, coronary artery disease, myocardial infarction.
  Symptomatic arrhythmias.
  Poorly controlled hypertension (diastolic greater than 110, systolic less than 160).
  History of congestive heart failure.
Respiratory
  Asthma/COPD requiring chronic medication or with acute exacerbation and progression within the past 6 months.
  History of major airway surgery or unusual airway anatomy.
  Upper or lower airway tumor or obstruction.
  History of chronic respiratory distress requiring home ventilatory assistance or monitoring.
Endocrine
  Insulin-dependent mellitus.
  Adrenal disorders.
  Active thyroid disease.
Neuromuscular
  History of seizure disorder or other significant CNS disease (e.g., multiple sclerosis).
  History of myopathy or other muscle disorders.
Hepatic
  Any active hepatobiliary disease or compromise.
Musculoskeletal
  Kyphosis or scoliosis causing functional compromise.
  Temporomandibular joint disorder.
  Cervical or thoracic spine injury.
Oncology
  Patients receiving chemotherapy.
  Other oncology process with significant physiologic residual or compromise.
Gastrointestinal
  Massive obesity (>140% ideal body weight).
  Hiatal hernia.
  Symptomatic gastroesophageal reflux.

* Reproduced with permission from Pasternak LR. Preoperative screening for ambulatory patients. *Anesthesiol Clin North America*. 2003;21(2):229–242. Copyright © Elsevier.

Table 12-2	**CONTRAINDICATIONS TO LAPAROSCOPIC SURGERY**

Absolute contraindications
  Shock
  IC Increased
  Severe myopia or retinal detachment
  Inadequate surgical skill or equipment
Relative contraindications
  Bullous emphysema or history of spontaneous pneumothorax
  Pregnancy
  Prolonged or new laparoscopic procedures

Ambulatory laparoscopic surgery

Ambulatory surgery is increasingly being practiced throughout North America. Newer anesthesia drugs and practices allow for faster recovery and improved perioperative care and minimal access techniques allow for a greater number of ambulatory procedures. Patients presenting for ambulatory surgery may have significant comorbid disease,[10,11] and while discharge criteria have been well formulated and practiced, there is little on patient selection criteria for ambulatory surgery.

Patients with pre-existing medical conditions presenting for ambulatory surgery should be stable and their disease should be optimally treated. They should have an escort to take them home and take care of them overnight, and they should understand instructions and be able to return for urgent care if their medical status deteriorates. Patients that are unlikely to be suitable for day-case surgery include patients who are classified as ASA Class 4, those who have had a recent MI (within last 30 days), moderate to severe angina (AHA Class III or IV angina) or heart failure symptoms (NYHA Class III or IV), patients who have severe morbid obesity (BMI >45 kg/m^2) or have severe sleep apnea, and those with sickle cell disease.[12] These patients usually require admission or overnight stay in a short-stay (23 hours) unit.

▌INTRAOPERATIVE MANAGEMENT

Despite the many advantages of minimal access surgery, there are significant physiologic changes and complications that are not necessarily seen with a laparotomy. Providing anesthesia for laparoscopic surgery can be challenging. While the effects of laparoscopy are usually well tolerated, patients with preexisting disease may experience more severe effects and have a limited capacity for compensation. Because these patients can deteriorate quickly in the event of a complication, recognition and timely management is required.

Physiologic changes during laparoscopy

The cardiovascular effects of the pneumoperitoneum appear to be somewhat phasic. Initially, the intraperitoneal insufflation of gas causes an increase in systemic vascular resistance (SVR), central venous pressure (CVP), and mean arterial pressure (MAP) along with a decrease in the cardiac index (CI).[13] Aortic compression contributes to an increase in SVR, while venous compression reduces flow through the inferior venous cava (IVC) and venous return to the heart, all of which can induce a decrease in cardiac output.[14] Within 10 minutes, the SVR gradually decreases and the CI returns towards normal. The cardiovascular changes are proportional to the intra-abdominal pressure (IAP) obtained: an insufflation pressure of 7 mm Hg has fewer hemodynamic effects than 15 mm Hg.[15] Patient position also influences the hemodynamic effects of laparoscopic surgery. For example, Trendelenburg position is associated with increased venous return, whereas reverse Trendelenburg further decreases venous return and CI. Carbon dioxide absorption from the CO_2 pneumoperitoneum can cause hypercapnia, which may further increase MAP, and raise heart rate, cardiac output, and plasma catecholamines,[13] in addition to increasing the risk of arrhythmias.

Bradyarrhythmias, from bradycardia to asystole, have occurred during laparoscopic surgery. They have been attributed to vagal stimulation from Veress needle or trocar insertion, peritoneal stretching from gas insufflation, fallopian tube stimulation by electrocautery, and venous air embolism.[6]

The cardiovascular changes seen with laparoscopic surgery may not always be predictable. Most patients tolerate laparoscopic surgery without significant hemodynamic alterations. Patients with hypovolemia, anemia or underlying cardiac disease, including coronary artery disease, poor ventricular function and regurgitant valvular disease may require particular attention to volume status, position, and IAP.

Regional blood flow is equally altered by laparoscopic surgery. As previously discussed, during abdominal insufflation there is an increase in the cerebral blood flow and ICP in direct relation to the IAP.[7] Compression of the IVC results in a rise of lumbar spinal pressure and subsequent decreased drainage from the lumbar plexus, and there is an elevated intrathoracic pressure from a celephad shift of the diaphragm with reduced venous drainage from the head.[13] Trendelenburg position further increases the ICP above the rise seen with pneumoperitoneum alone. Flow through the hepatoportal and splanchnic circulation and renal blood flow are also proportional to the IAP obtained. The potential for impaired splanchnic and renal circulation should be considered in critically ill patients.[13] Intra-abdominal insufflation of CO_2 is accompanied by a decrease in femoral vein flow, which is further worsened with a high IAP and reverse Trendelenburg position.[13] This alteration in lower extremity blood flow may increase the risk of venous thromboembolic disease.

Intraperitoneal insufflation of carbon dioxide has effects on pulmonary compliance and gas exchange. Trans-peritoneal absorption of CO_2 occurs within 10 minutes of the creation of the pneumoperitoneum, and its rate of absorption varies according to peritoneal cavity perfusion and duration of intraperitoneal insufflation.[13] Diffusion of CO_2 into the blood is also greater with extra-peritoneal gas insufflation. Despite increasing minute ventilation to normalize the changes in $PaCO_2$, refractory hypercapnia and acidosis can occur, particularly in ASA Class 3 and 4 patients.[16] An increase in minute ventilation and increased intrathoracic pressure from the pneumoperitoneum invariably lead to higher airway pressure, which can make ventilation and oxygenation of the obese patients or those with underlying respiratory disease quite difficult. The decreased pulmonary compliance seen with a cephalad shift of the diaphragm leads to intraoperative atelectasis and ventilation-perfusion mismatch, and can result in perioperative desaturation. The Trendelenburg position further accentuates the ventilatory effects of intraperitoneal gas insufflation, whereas a head-up position improves ventilation dynamics. Application of a constant positive end expiratory pressure (PEEP) of 5 cm H_2O has been shown to preserve PaO_2 during pneumoperitoneum, without significant hemodynamic consequences.[17]

Postoperatively, the changes to respiratory function return to normal, and lung function is better preserved than in a similar procedure completed via traditional laparotomy. Residual reductions in pulmonary function, both obstructive and restrictive, may be worse in upper abdominal laparoscopic surgery (laparoscopic cholecystectomy) than lower abdominal procedures (gynecologic laparoscopy) which is thought to be caused by reflex diaphragmatic inhibition.[13]

Choice of anesthetic

A wide variety of anesthetics have been used successfully for minimal access surgery. In most centres, general anesthesia is the preferred technique for patients undergoing laparoscopic surgery. Short-acting anesthetic agents allow for rapid recovery and quick OR turnover. General anesthesia with endotracheal intubation allows for administration of neuromuscular blocking agents and controlled ventilation during the pneumoperitoneum and head-down position, which allows for maintenance of normal $PaCO_2$, particularly during longer cases or those involving the upper abdomen. The laryngeal mask airway (LMA) has also been commonly used, particularly for short, day-case pelvic gynecologic laparoscopy. It is less traumatic than an endotracheal tube, and has not been shown to increase the risk of aspiration in patients who where considered low risk.[18] The LMA is most likely to be used with spontaneous ventilation, which appears to be safe in brief procedures with only a mild degree (e.g., 10 degree) of Trendelenburg.[18]

Regional anesthesia, on the other hand, offers many advantages over general anesthesia, including quicker recovery, decreased postoperative nausea and vomiting (PONV) and shorter postoperative stay.[19] However, this approach requires a cooperative patient, low IAP (to reduce pain and ventilatory disturbances), a minimal head-down position, and a rapid and gentle surgical technique.[6] Spontaneous breathing may become difficult for procedures that require steep Trendelenburg, large pneumoperitoneum, or a complex surgical technique (multiple port sites, significant organ handling, or prolonged time). In practice, regional anesthesia or general anesthesia with a laryngeal mask and spontaneous ventilation are reserved mostly for laparoscopic tubal ligations.[19]

Complications

Complications that are unique to laparoscopic procedures are connected to the intraperitoneal insufflation of gas, surgical instrumentation and patient positioning.[2] The incidence of complications depends on the type of procedure and training and experience of the surgeon performing the procedure—increased experience decreases the number of bowel injuries and also changes the approach to the management of complications with a reduced rate of conversion to laparotomy.[20] The complication rate is reported to be up to four times higher in surgeons having performed less than 100 laparoscopic procedures.[2] When examining the data from laparoscopic hysterectomy, injury to the bladder occurs in less than 2%

of cases, to the ureter in less than 0.5%, to bowel in less than 0.5%, and vascular injury in less than 0.1%.[21] These rates are all higher than those cited for hysterectomy via laparotomy. In a large study looking at complications following laparoscopic hysterectomy, major complications occurred in 2.2% of cases, with one postoperative death (0.002%) from a massive pulmonary embolus.[22] Comparatively, the overall mortality rate for laparoscopic cholecystectomy has declined to less than 0.6%, and the overall complication rate to approximately 2.5%.[2]

Extraperitoneal gas insufflation

Inadvertent blind misplacement of the Veress needle can lead to it being positioned in a vessel, subcutaneous tissue, viscus, omentum, mesentery, or retroperitoneum.

Subcutaneous emphysema, from the preperitonal insufflation of gas, can be identified by crepitus over the abdominal wall, which can then extend to the groin or towards the chest wall and neck. The area for CO_2 absorption increases, which leads to a persistent hypercapnia despite increased minute ventilation, and can cause a significant respiratory acidosis. In fact, a rising end-tidal CO_2 is an early sign of extra-peritoneal gas insufflation.[23] The incidence rates for subcutaneous emphysema during laparoscopy vary from 0.5% to 2.4%, and risk factors include longer operative time and the use of six or more operative ports.[24] Nitrous oxide should be discontinued as it may further expand the emphysema, but in most cases, no specific treatment is required as the subcutaneous emphysema resolves after the abdomen is deflated.[2] Subcutaneous air that has tracked to the neck and face may compromise the airway of an extubated patient, and may also extend to the thorax, causing a pneumothorax or pneumomediastinum. It may be prudent to perform a chest X-ray or CT in patients with cervical emphysema, in order to rule out intrathoracic extension.

Pneumothorax, penumomediastinum, and pneumopericardium

Extension of subcutaneous emphysema can lead to air in the thorax or mediastinum.[25] Alternatively, the gas can enter the thorax through a tear in the visceral peritoneum, around the esophagus during surgical dissection, or by a congenital defect in the diaphragm.[2] Spontaneous rupture of pre-existing lung bullae can also result in pneumothorax.

A pneumothorax can be aymptomatic, but can also present with desaturation, increased airway pressures, hypotension and even cardiac arrest.[26] Although a rare complication, it is potentially life-threatening and requires early diagnosis and immediate treatment. The management of a pneumothorax during laparoscopic surgery includes deflating the pneumoperitoneum, continuing supportive treatment, confirming the diagnosis by chest X-ray (if patient is stable), and treating according to size and effect of the pneumothorax.[2] A large or hemodynamically compromising pneumothorax requires immediate decompression and placement of a chest tube. Conversion to a laparotomy may be necessary.

The mechanisms of pneumomediastinum are thought to be similar to those of pneumothorax, and they can cause hemodynamic instability and bronchial obstruction.[2] Pneumopericardium can occur when the gas is forced into the mediastinum and pericardium via the IVC. Both complications are relatively rare, and the release of the penumoperitoneum is usually all that is required for treatment.

Gas embolism

Vascular air embolism (VAE) is the entrainment of gas into venous or arterial vessels, which produces systemic effects. The incidence is unknown, as many cases of VAE are subclinical and go undetected. Both the volume of gas entrainment and the rate of accumulation determine the morbidity and mortality from VAE, and the adult lethal volume has been described as between 200 and 300 mL.[27] The volume and rate of accumulation depend on the size of the vessel as well as the pressure gradient. For instance, negative pressure gradients, such as a craniotomy in a sitting position, and positive pressure insufflation of gas, as with laparoscopic procedures, have a risk of VAE. Laparoscopic procedures are thought to have a relatively high risk of VAE (greater than 25%), with gas entrainment through open vascular channels from surgical dissection rather than simply a complication of intraperitoneal insufflation.[27]

Gas bubbles in the pulmonary vasculature lead to pulmonary hypertension, systemic inflammatory response syndrome and pulmonary edema. Signs and symptoms can include hypoxia, decreased end-tidal CO_2, increased airway pressures, arrhythmias, ECG changes suggestive of cardiac ischemia, and hypotension. A large volume of air embolism (5 mL/kg) can cause an airlock scenario, with complete outflow obstruction from the right ventricle, and cardiovascular collapse and even death.[27] Because CO_2 is more soluble in blood than air, a greater volume of carbon dioxide embolism can be tolerated when compared to an air embolism. In addition, rapid absorption of the CO_2 embolus leads to rapid reversal of hemodynamic impairment.[2] A patent foramen ovale (PFO), which occurs in 20% of the adult population, allows the VAE to enter the systemic circulation and can result in a stroke or cerebral edema.

A high index of suspicion and appropriate monitoring may allow for early detection and management of CO_2 embolism. In order to stop further entrainment of gas, insufflation of CO_2 should be immediately discontinued and pneumoperitoneum released, and the patient should be placed in a reverse Trendelenburg position. Oxygenation should be maximized and volume of embolus reduced by placing the patient on 100% oxygen and discontinuing nitrous oxide, if used.[27] Hyperventilation allows for more rapid elimination of CO_2. If an airlock is suspected, placing the patient in a partial left lateral decubitus position and aspiration of the emboli from the right atrium via an in situ central access catheter may improve hemodynamics.[27] Chest compressions may improve forwards blood flow by breaking up larger gas bubbles and dispersing them into the pulmonary vessels.[27] Inotropes and vasopressors may be required for ongoing hemodynamic support, and hyperbaric oxygen has been successfully used in cases of cerebral arterial gas embolism.[2] A differential diagnosis for cardiovascular collapse during laparoscopic surgery is detailed in Table 12-3.

Vascular injuries

Vascular injury can occur during insertion of the Veress needle or trocar, or can occur during surgical dissection. In the gynecologic literature, the overall incidence of vascular injury varies quite a bit, from 0.64% to 1.1%,[2,28] which is somewhat higher than that found in gastrointestinal and urologic laparoscopic procedures, where the incidence of major vascular

Table 12-3	DIFFERENTIAL DIAGNOSIS OF SUDDEN CARDIOVASCULAR COLLAPSE DURING LAPAROSCOPY*
Profound vasovagal reaction	
Cardiac arrhythmias	
Excessive IAPs	
Acute hemorrhage	
Myocardial ischemia	
Tension pneumothorax	
Severe respiratory acidosis	
Venous gas embolism	
Cardiac tamponade	
Anaphylaxis	

* Data adapted from Joshi GP. Complications of laparoscopy. *Anesthesiol Clin North America*. 2001; 19(1):89–105.

injuries is 0.03% to 0.06%.[2] The incidence of vascular injury decreases with surgical experience.

Insertion of the Veress needle or trocar into major vessels such as the aorta, common iliac vessels, or inferior vena cava has been reported.[2] Trocars can also cause injury to vessels of the abdominal wall, or the mesenteric vessels, resulting in hemorrhage or hematoma formation. Most abdominal wall bleeding is self-limited, but hemostasis to persistent bleeding has been performed using sutures, coagulation, and tamponade with a balloon from a Foley catheter.[29] Placement of the trocar through a minilaparotomy incision and subsequent secondary trocars with transillumination and under direct vision should reduce associated vessel injury. Return of blood from the Veress needle or trocar identifies injury to a major vessel, but the hemorrhage can be concealed and may present as unexplained hypotension. There is often a delay of diagnosis when the bleeding has reached the retroperitoneal space. A Veress needle or trocar placed into a vessel should be left in situ to avoid further bleeding and to help identify the site of injury. Immediate laparotomy should be performed to control the bleeding, using packs or digital pressure, and to repair the injury.[2] Early consultation from a vascular surgeon is recommended. Massive intraoperative hemorrhage requires ongoing resuscitation with fluid and blood products, and patients may require postoperative care in a monitored setting.

Vascular injury can also occur during operative laparoscopy, unrelated to trocar or Veress needle injury. Injury may occur during surgical dissection or laceration with unipolar electrosurgery, sharp scissors, or CO_2 laser.[30] Laparoscopic lymph node dissection in particular may have an increased risk of vascular injury,[28,30] as it is by definition a perivascular dissection. Laparoscopic repair can be attempted by experienced surgeons,[28] but control of bleeding should not be delayed. Conversion to laparotomy may be required.

Theoretically, there is a concern of gas embolism when venous injury occurs. This complication is most likely when the Veress needle or trocar is inserted directly into the vessel, as a bleeding injured vein is less likely to suck up gas.[30]

Nerve injury

Injuries to nerves during laparoscopic surgery can occur as a result of surgical complications, or because of the patient position. Peripheral nerve injuries occur in approximately one in a 1000 to one in 350 anesthetics, with the ulnar nerve being involved in most cases.[31] Injury to the brachial plexus can occur as a result of prolonged direct pressure from shoulder rests (which prevent the patient from slipping off the table when in steep head-down position), or as a result of stretching of the brachial plexus with the arm in excessive abduction.[28] Improper use of leg stirrups with the patient in the lithotomy position may expose the common peroneal nerve or saphenous nerve to injury.[29] During prolonged laparoscopic surgery, careful positioning is necessary to avoid nerve compression injury.

Trendelenburg position

The cardiovascular and respiratory complications of Trendelenburg position have previously been discussed. Such positioning increases CVP, decreases lung volumes and increases airway ventilation pressures, and increases intracranial and intraocular pressures. When Trendelenburg is combined with prolonged hypotension and the intraoperative administration of large quantities of fluid, there is a risk of compromise to the ocular circulation.[32] The Trendelenburg position can cause venous distension of the upper body and swelling of the tongue and face. Also, combined with reduced venous outflow from the head and neck caused by pneumoperitoneum, postextubation respiratory failure from laryngeal edema has occurred.[33]

Brachial plexus injuries may occur as a result of shoulder braces placed close to the neck to prevent change in position during steep head-down tilt. Since Trendelenburg positions the operative site in the pelvis above the heart, a pressure gradient is created and the risk of venous air embolism may be increased.

POSTOPERATIVE CARE

Although laparoscopic surgery results in less postoperative pain than a laparotomy, postoperative pain can still be significant. In addition, the risk of PONV after laparoscopic gynecological surgery is relatively high. Both pain and PONV need to be controlled for ambulatory patients. For advanced laparoscopic gynecological surgery, particularly for cancer patients, an additional consideration is prevention of venous thromboembolism (VTE).

Postoperative pain control

Almost all patients who undergo minimal access surgery still have pain symptoms 24 hours postoperatively, with neck and shoulder pain and abdominal pain being the most common.[18] Half of outpatients complain of incisional pain after laparoscopic surgery, which is twice the overall incidence of all pain complaints in outpatients.[6] Acute pain after laparoscopic surgical techniques can be complex, and includes incisional pain, visceral pain from pelvic inflammation and scapular pain secondary to peritoneal insufflation. Prevention and treatment of postoperative pain includes the use of local anesthetics, nonsteroidal anti-inflammatory drugs (NSAIDs), opioids, and other adjuncts, as well as various surgical techniques.

Local anesthesia

Infiltration of the laparoscopy portals with local anesthetic has been shown, in laparoscopic cholecystectomy, to reduce pain scores for up to 24 hours after surgery.[34] Preemptive infiltration of local anesthetic for inguinal herniorrhaphy also reduces postoperative analgesic requirements. Patients undergoing noncancer laparoscopic gynecological surgery had a longer delay before requesting their first analgesic and experienced significantly less pain 24 hours postoperatively when 0.5% bupivacaine was infiltrated at the surgical site before incision, compared to those infiltrated at skin closure and those receiving placebo.[35] This would suggest that preemptive infiltration of the portal sites before skin incision offers better pain control in the postoperative period, perhaps because the local anesthetic blocks the sensitization of peripheral pain receptors to tissue damage. However, a similar study in day-case minor laparoscopic gynecological procedures comparing pre- or postincision bupivacaine portal infiltration to normal saline did not show any significant difference in mean pain scores or incisional pain between the treatment groups or with the placebo group.[36]

Intraperitoneal instillation of local anesthetic has been shown to have variable results when applied to laparacopic cholecystectomy.[34] A large randomized-control trial comparing intraperitoneal instillation of 20 mL of bupivacaine (0.5% with 1:200,000 epinephrine), ropivacaine (0.75%) or normal saline for major laparoscopic gynecological surgery demonstrated that opioid analgesic requirements were significantly decreased in the local anesthetic groups, both immediately after surgery and in the first 24 hours postoperatively.[37] In addition, the incidence of PONV was significantly reduced for both treatment groups as compared to placebo. When bupivacaine was combined with the infusion of intraperitoneal Hartmann's solution to reduce the incidence of postoperative adhesions after major laparoscopic gynecological procedures, there was no difference in postoperative pain scores or analgesic consumption compared to placebo.[38]

Epidural local anesthetics work by blocking afferent nerve activity at the spinal cord level, and its effect on postoperative analgesia and outcomes in major surgical procedures has been well established.[39] Postoperative recovery using epidural analgesia after laparoscopic colonic surgery has been shown to be superior to systemic opioids, with improved pain relief, earlier mobilization and discharge, and a reduction in postoperative ileus.[40,41] Few studies have looked at epidural use for postoperative pain control in major laparoscopic gynecological surgery. Initiation of an epidural with lidocaine and morphine prior to skin incision improves postoperative pain scores in the first 12 hours after laparoscopic radical hysterectomy for cervical cancer, compared to starting the epidural only after skin closure.[42] In addition, improvement of immune function was observed intraoperatively, and the authors speculated that this could lead to an improvement in long-term cancer survival.

Nonsteroidal anti-inflammatory drugs

NSAIDs modulate the local inflammatory response by inhibiting cyclooxygenase both in the spinal cord and the periphery, to reduce prostaglandin synthesis. Acetaminophen inhibits the synthesis of prostaglandins in the central nervous system.[34] Both NSAIDs and acetaminophen have been shown to speed up recovery and reduce opioid analgesic use after lapararoscopy and other minor surgical procedures. The optimal use of NSAIDs and acetaminophen is obtained by continuous prophylactic use for 3 to 4 days postoperatively, particularly when used in combination with each other.[34] In a study treating patients with a short course of celecoxib after ambulatory laparoscopic surgery, mean pain scores and need for analgesics, both at 24 and 48 hours postoperatively, were significantly reduced compared to placebo, and the quality of recovery was improved with celecoxib.[43] When ketorolac was combined with dextromethorphan (an N-methyl-D-aspartate receptor antagonist) preoperatively for patients undergoing laparoscopic-assisted vaginal hysterectomy, patients had improved pain scores and reduced opioid analgesic requirements compared to placebo.[44]

Short courses of NSAIDs and acetaminophen postoperatively are well tolerated and have good safety profile.[6] They provide superior analgesia and their opioid-sparing properties may reduce the incidence of nausea, vomiting, sedation and pruritus.

Opioids

Opioid analgesics are obviously effective in treating pain after laparoscopic procedures, but certain routes of administration may be superior to others.

Patient-controlled analgesia (PCA) IV opioids have been studied for total abdominal hysterectomy, but not for major or advanced laparoscopic gynecological surgery. In a recent study comparing the analgesic requirements in patients undergoing total laparoscopic hysterectomy (TLH) to those submitted to vaginal hysterectomy, patients undergoing TLH required approximately 50% less postoperative PCA IV opioids.[45]

Controlled-release (CR) narcotics may provide better analgesia in outpatient laparoscopic surgical procedures. Given as a premedication, oxycodone CR has been shown to reduce pain and the incidence of PONV after ambulatory laparoscopic tubal ligation, but not after minor laparoscopic gynecologic day-case surgery.[46,47] Further studies are required to define the optimal opioid analgesics for patients undergoing major or advanced gynecological minimal access surgery.

Analgesic adjuncts

Preoperative steroid administration attenuates the postoperative inflammatory activation, and its analgesic effect is provided by decreasing products of cyclooxygenase and lipoxygenase pathways.[34] A single dose of IV dexamethasone (8 mg) given before laparoscopic cholecystectomy reduced postoperative pain and opioid requirements by approximately 50% compared to placebo, in addition to improvement of PONV.[48] Similarly, a single intraoperative dose of IV dexamethasone (8 mg) improved both PONV and analgesic requirements after gynecological laparoscopic surgery, compared to both placebo and a lower dose of dexamethasone.[49] Obviously, there are concerns about a possible association of steroids with impaired wound healing, postoperative infection, and other complications, but two meta-analyses have not indicated that a single dose of dexamethasone increased postoperative complications.[34]

Gabapentin, originally used as an anticonvulsant, also works centrally to decrease the release of monoamine neurotransmitters. It has been shown to reduce postoperative pain and opioid consumption after abdominal hysterectomy, major orthopedic surgery, and laparoscopic cholecystectomy.[34] Its use for laparoscopic gynecological surgery, however, has not yet been studied.

Surgical technique

Shoulder pain is one of the most common complaints of pain in the first 24 hours after laparoscopic surgery. The severity of the pain is directly related to the volume of residual gas: the greater the residual gas volume (calculated from radiologic imaging), the greater the amount of shoulder pain.[50] A study of 161 women undergoing minor laparoscopic gynecological procedures showed that an intraperitoneal drain placed at the end of the surgery that remained in situ for 4 hours reduced the frequency of postoperative shoulder pain and the postoperative analgesic requirements compared to a sham drain.[51]

Distension of the abdomen alone causes pain, and one study has shown that using gas insufflation pressures of 7 to 9 mm Hg reduced postoperative shoulder pain after laparoscopic cholecystectomy compared with higher insufflation pressures (12–14 mm Hg).[34] Using heated or humidified CO_2 for intraperitoneal insufflation has not been shown to have any effect on postoperative pain scores or analgesic requirements after laparoscopic gynecological surgery.[52]

Since the pain after laparoscopic surgical procedures has multiple etiologies, it makes sense that a combination of analgesic methods will be most effective. Simple measures, such as evacuating the insufflated CO_2, intraperitoneal instillation and preincision infiltration of a long-acting local anesthetic to portal sites, intraoperative administration of dexamethasone, and perioperative use of NSAIDs and acetaminophen, may reduce postoperative pain safely and effectively. With major and advanced laparoscopic gynecological surgery, it may be of additional benefit to add a controlled-release narcotic or gabapentin preoperatively, and extend its use into the postoperative period. High-quality studies are needed in laparoscopic gynecological surgery to provide evidence for the optimal multimodal analgesic regimen.

VTE prophylaxis

The lithotomy and Trendelenburg positions used for advanced laparoscopic gynecological surgery impede blood flow in the lower extremities and result in venous stasis. High IAPs can increase the likelihood for deep vein thrombosis (DVT) and pulmonary embolism (PE), as there is compression of the femoral veins and a reduction in femoral vein flow velocity.[2] The risk of VTE and need for prophylaxis in patients having undergone minimal access surgery is poorly defined: minimal tissue trauma and early ambulation associated with laparoscopic procedures may outweigh intraoperative venous stasis.

Venous thromboembolic complications following laparoscopic cholecystectomy are relatively low: DVT, 0.02%; pulmonary embolism, 0.06%; fatal pulmonary embolism, 0.02%; and mortality, 0.1%.[53] In 266 patients having laparoscopy for noncancer related procedures, none were diagnosed with compressive ultrasound detected DVT or clinically relevant VTE after a 2-week follow-up, despite lack of VTE prophylaxis.[54] In a larger study with 1265 major and advanced laparoscopic gynecologic procedures (hysterectomy accounted for 29%), postoperative VTE was diagnosed in 0.4%.[55] In recent large, multicentre studies, the risk of VTE in laparoscopic noncancer gastrointestinal procedures is around 0.3%, and in laparoscopic radical prostatectomy for prostate cancer, the risk of VTE is closer to 0.5%.[56,57] These rates for DVT are all significantly lower than the 15% to 40% risk of DVT after major open gastrointestinal, urologic or gynecologic surgery.[58]

Several factors increase the risk of VTE following gynecologic surgery, including malignancy, older age, prior pelvic radiation therapy, compression of major pelvic veins by an intraabdominal mass and venous trauma from pelvic lymph node dissection. Major and advanced laparoscopic gynecological may also have prolonged surgical times with significant venous stasis from the penumoperitoneum. The American College of Chest Physicians has recommended that thromboprophylaxis should be provided for patients undergoing laparoscopic gynecologic procedures in whom additional VTE risk factors are present (Table 12-4). They recommend the use of at least one of the following: low-dose unfractionated heparin, low-molecular-weight heparin, intermittent pneumatic compression

Table 12-4   RISK FACTORS FOR VENOUS THROMBOEMBOLISM*
Immobility, paresis
Malignancy
Cancer therapy (hormonal, chemotherapy, or radiotherapy)
Previous VTE
Increased age
Pregnancy and the postpartum period
Estrogen-containing oral contraception or HRT
Selective estrogen receptor modulators
Acute medical illness
Heart or respiratory failure
Inflammatory bowel disease
Nephrotic syndrome, paroxysmal norturnal hemoglobinuria
Myeloproliferative disorders
Obesity
Smoking
Varicose veins
Inherited or acquired thrombophilia

* Adapted with permission from Seventh ACCP Conference on Antithrombotic and Thrombolytic Therapy. Prevention of venous thromboembolism. *Chest.* 2004;126(3):338S–400S.

devices, or graduated compression stockings.[58] Prophylaxis should continue until discharge from hospital, and may be considered for a further 2 to 4 weeks for those considered particularly high risk.

Discharge criteria for ambulatory laparoscopic gynecological surgery

As day-case surgery continues to expand, side effects which may be considered minor in the inpatient can contribute to unexpected admissions and increased costs. PONV is a common postoperative complication, with an incidence of up to 77% after gynecologic laparoscopy, and is the most common cause (61%) for unplanned admission in ambulatory surgery.[59] Other major reasons for unscheduled admissions after day-case gynecological laparoscopy include pain, urinary retention and surgical concerns. Several pharmacologic therapies have been shown to be effective for preventing PONV after laproscopic gynecological surgery: serotonin antagonists (ondansetron, granisetron, dolasetron), dexamethasone, droperidol, haloperidol, and propofol infusions.[6,49,60,61] Avoidance of nitrous oxide and narcotics has also been suggested.

Discharge from the ambulatory surgical unit requires that a patient have sufficiently recovered to leave under the supervision of a caregiver. Criteria for safe discharge from the hospital include stable vital signs, adequate level of consciousness, independence with dressing and ambulating, ability to void and tolerate oral fluids, and minimal pain and nausea.[62] In addition, the patient should have written instructions for the postoperative period. The Postanesthetic Discharge Scoring System (PADS) has been used to determine when patients can be discharged home safely.[63] Most patients can be discharged 1 to 2 hours after surgery.

CONCLUSION

Laparoscopic gynecologic surgery aims to minimize the traumatic surgical process while accomplishing sometimes complex and life-saving procedures. With control of pain and PONV, patients recover quickly and can be discharged home earlier than with a similar "open" technique.

Intraoperative complications of laparoscopic surgery are because of the physiologic changes associated to the intraperitoneal insufflation of gas and patient positioning, as well as traumatic injuries from trocars or surgical dissection. Quick diagnosis and management of complications provide the best patient outcomes. General anesthesia with controlled ventilation is the preferred anesthetic technique, and patients with significant comorbidity require careful perioperative monitoring.

REFERENCES

1. Gonzalez R, Smith CD. McClusky DA. et al. Laparoscopic approach reduces likelihood of perioperative complications in patients undergoing adrenalectomy. *Am Surg.* 2004;70(8):668-674.

2. Joshi GP. Complications of laparoscopy. *Anesthesiol Clin North America.* 2001; 19(1):89-105.

3. Klopfenstein CE, Forster A, Van Gessel E. Anesthetic assessment in an outpatient consultation clinic reduces preoperative anxiety. *Can J Anesth.* 2000;47(6):511-515.

4. Pasternak LR. Preoperative screening for ambulatory patients. *Anesthesiol Clin North America.* 2003;21(2):229-242.

5. ACC/AHA Guideline. ACC/AHA Guidelines on perioperative cardiovascular evaluation and care for noncardiac surgery. *Circulation.* 2007;116(17):e418-e49.

6. Gerges FJ, Kanazi GE. Jabbour-khoury SI. Anesthesia for laparoscopy: A review. *J Clin Anesth.* 2006;18(1):67-78.

7. Mobbs RJ, Yang MO. The dangers of diagnostic laparoscopy in the head injured patient. *J Clinc Neurosci.* 2002;9(5):592-593.

8. Ravaoherisoa J, Meyer P, Afriat R, et al. Laparoscopic surgery in a patient with ventriculoperitoneal shunt: Monitoring of shunt function with transcranial Doppler. *Br J Anaesth.* 2004;92(3):434-437.

9. Stepp K, Falcone T. Laparoscopy in the second trimester of pregnancy. *Obstet Gynecol Clin North America.* 2004;31(3):485-496.

10. Chung F, Mezei G, Tong D. Pre-existing medical conditions as predictors of adverse events in day-case surgery. *Br J Anaesth.* 1999;83(2):262-270.

11. Chung F, Mezei G, Tong D. Adverse events in ambulatory surgery: A comparison between elderly and younger patients. *Can J Anesth.* 1999;46(4):309-321.

12. Friedman Z, Chung F, Wong DT. Ambulatory surgery adult patient selection criteria: A survey of Canadian anesthesiologists. *Can J Anesth.* 2004;51(5):437-443.

13. O'Malley C, Cunningham AJ. Physiologic changes during laparoscopy. *Anesthesiol Clin North America.* 2001;19(1):1-19.

14. Ortega AE, Richman MF, Hernandez M, et al. Inferior vena caval blood flow and cardiac hemodynamics during carbon dioxide pneumoperitoneum. *Surgl Endosc.* 1996;10(9):920-924.

15. Dexter SP, Vucevic M, Gibson J, et al. Hemodynamic consequences of high- and low-pressure capnoperitoneum during laparoscopic cholecystectomy. *Surg Endosc.* 1999;13(4):376-381.

16. Wittgen CM, Andrus CH, Fitzgerald SD, et al. Analysis of the hemodynamic and ventilatory effects of laparoscopic cholecystectomy. *Arch Surg.* 1991;126(8):997-1000.

17. Meininger D, Byhahn C, Mierdl S, et al. Positive end-expiratory pressure improves arterial oxygenation during prolonged pneumoperitoneum. *Acta Anaesthesiol Scand.* 2005;49(6):778-783.

18. Smith I. Anesthesia for laparoscopy with emphasis on outpatient laparoscopy. *Anesthesiol Clin North America.* 2001;19(1):21-41.

19. Collins LM, Vaghadia H. Regional anesthesia for laparoscopy. *Anesthesiol Clin North America.* 2001;19(1):43-55.

20. Chapron C, Querleu D, Bruhat MA, et al. Surgical complications of diagnostic and operative gynaecological laparoscopy: A series of 29,966 cases. *Hum Reprod.* 1998;13(4):867-872.

21. Parker WH. Total laparoscopic hysterectomy and laparoscopic supracervical hysterectomy. *Obstet Gynecol Clin North Am.* 2004;31(3):523-537.

22. Harkki-Siren P, Sjoberg J, Kurki T. Major complications of laparoscopy: A follow-up Finnish study. *Obstet Gynecol.* 1999;94(1):94-98.

23. Pearce DJ. Respiratory acidosis and subcutaneous emphysema during laparoscopic cholecystectomy. *Can J Anesth.* 1994;41(4):314-316.

24. Murdock CM, Wolff AJ, Van Geem T. Risk factors for hypercarbia, subcutaneous emphysema, penumothorax, and pneumomediastinum during laparoscopy. *Obstet Gynecol.* 2000;95:704-709.

25. Stern JA, Nadler RB. Pneumothorax masked by subcutaneous emphysema after laparoscopic nephrectomy. *J Endourol.* 2004;18(5):457-458.

26. Mangar D, Kirchhoff GT, Leal JJ, et al. Penumothorax during laparoscopic Nissen fundoplication. *Can J Anesth.* 1994;41(9):854-856.

27. Mirski MA, Lele AV, Fitzsimmons L, et al. Diagnosis and treatment of vascular air embolism. *Anesthesiology.* 2007;106(1):164-177.

28. Querleu D, Leblanc E, Cartron G, et al. Audit of preoperative and early complications of laparoscopic lymph node dissection in 1000 gynecologic cancer patients. *Am J Obstet Gynecol.* 2006;195(5):1287-1292.

29. Li TC, Saravelos H, Richmond M. et al. Complications of laparoscopic pelvic surgery: Recognition, management and prevention. *Hum Reprod Update.* 1997;3(5):505-515.

30. Nezhat C, Childers J, Nezhat F, et al. Major retroperitoneal vascular injury laparoscopic surgery. *Hum Reprod.* 1997;12(3):480-483.

31. Sawyer RJ, Richmond MN, Hickey JD, et al. Peripheral nerve injuries associated with anesthesia. *Anaesthesia.* 2000;55(10):980-991.

32. Roth S, Nunez R, Schreider BD. Unexplained visual loss after lumbar spine fusion. *J Neurosurg Anesthesiol.* 1997;9(4):346-348.

33. Phing SV, Koh LK. Anaesthesia for robotic-assisted radical prostatectomy: Considerations for laparoscopy in the Trendelenburg position. *Anaesth Intensive Care.* 2007;35(2):281-285.

34. Bisgaard T. Analgesic treatment after laparoscopic cholecystectomy: A critical assessment of the evidence. *Anesthesiology.* 2006;104(4):835-846.

35. Ke RW, Portera SG, Bagous W, et al. A randomized, double-blinded trial of preemptive analgesia in laparoscopy. *Obstet Gynecol.* 1998;92(6):972-975.

36. Fong SY, Pavy TJG, Yeo ST, et al. Assessment of wound infiltration with bupivacaine in women undergoing day-case gynecological laparoscopy. *Reg Anesth Pain Med.* 2001;26(2):131–136.

37. Goldstein A, Grimault P, Henique A, et al. Preventing postoperative pain by local anesthetic instillation after laparoscopic gynecologic surgery: A placebo-controlled comparison of bupivacaine and ropivacaine. *Anesth Analg.* 2000; 91(2):403–407.

38. Shaw IC, Stevens J, Krishnamurthy S. The influence of intraperitoneal bupivacaine on pain following major laparoscopic gynaecological procedures. *Anaesthesia.* 2001;56(11):1041–1044.

39. Liu SS, Wu CL. Effect of postoperative analgesia on major postoperative complications: A systematic update of the evidence. *Anesth Analg.* 2007;104(3):689–702.

40. Bardam L, Funch-Jensen P, Jensen P, et al. Recovery after laparoscopic colonic surgery with epidural analgesia, and early oral nutrition and mobilization. *Lancet.* 1995;345(8952):763–764.

41. Senagore AJ, Whalley D, Delaney CP, et al. Epidural anesthesia-analgesia shortens length of stay after laparoscopic segmental colectomy for benign pathology. *Surgery.* 2001;129(6):672–676.

42. Hong J-Y, Lim KT. Effect of preemptive epidural analgesia on cytokine response and postoperative pain in laparoscopic radical hysterectomy for cervical cancer. *Reg Anesth Pain Medi.* 2008;33(1):44–51.

43. White PF, Sacan O, Tufanogullari B. *et al.* Effect of short-term postoperative celecoxib administration on patient outcome after outpatient laparoscopic surgery. Canadian Journal of Anesthesia. 54(5):342–348, 2007.

44. Lu CH, Liu JY, Lee MS, et al. Preoperative cotreatment with dextromethorphan and ketorolac provides an enhancement of pain relief after laparoscopic-assisted vaginal hysterectomy. *Clin J Pain.* 2006;22(9):799–804.

45. Nascimento MC, Kelley A, Martitsch C, et al. Postoperative analgesic requirements: Total laparoscopic hysterectomy versus vaginal hysterectomy. *Aust N Z J Obstet Gynaecol.* 2005;45(2):140–143.

46. Reuben SS, Steinberg RB, Maciolek H, et al. Preoperative administration of controlled-release oxycodone for the management of pain after ambulatory laparoscopic tubal ligation surgery. *J Clin Anesth.* 2002;14(3):223–227.

47. Jokela R, Ahonen J, Valjus M, et al. Premedication with controlled-release oxycodone does not improve management of postoperative pain after day-case gynaecological laparoscopic surgery. *Br J Anaesth.* 2007;98(2):255–260.

48. Bisgaard T, Klarskov B, Kehlet H, et al. Preoperative dexamethasone improves surgical outcome after laparoscopic cholecystectomy: A randomized double-blind placebo-controlled trial. *Ann Surg.* 2003;238(5):651–660.

49. Fujii Y, Nakayama M. Dexamethasone for reduction of nausea, vomiting and analgesic use after gynecological laparoscopic surgery. *Int J Gynaecol Obstet.* 2008;100(1):27–30.

50. Jackson SA, Laurence AS, Hill JC. Does post-laparoscopy pain relate to residual carbon dioxide? *Anaesthesia.* 1996;51(5):485–487.

51. Abbott J, Hawe J, Srivastava P, et al. Intraperitoneal gas drain to reduce pain after laparoscopy: Randomized masked trial. *Obstet Gynecol.* 2001;98(1):97–100.

52. Kissler S, Hass M, Strohmeier R, et al. Effect of humidified and heated CO_2 during gynecologic laparoscopic surgery on analgesics and postoperative pain. *J Am Assoc Gynecol Laparosc.* 2004;11(4):473–477.

53. Bergqvist D, Lowe L. Venous thromboembolism in patients undergoing laparoscopic and arthroscopic surgery and in leg casts. *Arch Intern Med.* 2002; 162(19):2173–2176.

54. Ageno W. The incidence of venous thromboembolism following gynecologic laparoscopy: A multicenter, prospective cohort study. *J Thromb and Haemost.* 2007;5(3):503–506.

55. Johnston K. Major complications arising from 1265 operative laparoscopic cases: A prospective review from a single centre. *J Minim Invasive Gynecol.* 2007;14(3):339–344.

56. Nguyen NT. Laparoscopic surgery is associated with a lower incidence of venous thromboembolism compared with open surgery. *Ann Surg.* 2007;246(6):1021–1027.

57. Secin FP. Multi-institutional study of symptomatic deep venous thrombosis and pulmonary embolism in prostate cancer patients undergoing laparoscopic or robot-assisted laparoscopic radical prostatectomy. *Eur Urol.* 2008;53(1):134–145.

58. Seventh ACCP Conference on Antithrombotic and Thrombolytic Therapy. Prevention of venous thromboembolism. *Chest.* 2004;126(3):338S–400S.

59. Hedayati B, Fear S. Hospital admission after day-case gynaecological laparoscopy. *Br J Anaesth.* 1999;83(5):776–779.

60. Wang TF, Liu YH, Chu CC, et al. Low-dose haloperidol prevents post-operative nausea and vomiting after ambulatory laparoscopic surgery. *Acta Anaesthesiol Scand.* 2008;52(2):280–284.

61. Cameron D, Gan TJ. Management for postoperative nausea and vomiting in ambulatory surgery. *Anesthesiol Clin North Am.* 2003;21(2):347–365.

62. Marshall SI, Chung F. Discharge criteria and complications after ambulatory surgery. *Anesth Analg.* 1999;88(3):508–517.

63. Chung F, Chan V, Ong D. A postanesthetic discharge scoring system for home readiness after ambulatory surgery. *J Clin Anesth.* 1995;7(6):500–506.

Index

Note: Page numbers followed by f indicate figure and followed by t indicate table.